Practice Management: Successfully Guiding Your Group into the Future

Editors

AMR E. ABOULEISH
STANLEY W. STEAD

ANESTHESIOLOGY CLINICS

www.anesthesiology.theclinics.com

Consulting Editor
LEE A. FLEISHER

June 2018 • Volume 36 • Number 2

ELSEVIER

1600 John F. Kennedy Boulevard • Suite 1800 • Philadelphia, Pennsylvania, 19103-2899

http://www.theclinics.com

ANESTHESIOLOGY CLINICS Volume 36, Number 2
June 2018 ISSN 1932-2275, ISBN-13: 978-0-323-58390-9

Editor: Colleen Dietzler
Developmental Editor: Kristen Helm

Anesthesiology Clinics (ISSN 1932-2275) is published quarterly by Elsevier Inc., 360 Park Avenue South, New York, NY 10010-1710. Months of issue are March, June, September, and December. Periodicals postage paid at New York, NY and at additional mailing offices. Subscription prices are $100.00 per year (US student/resident), $346.00 per year (US individuals), $437.00 per year (Canadian individuals), $657.00 per year (US institutions), $830.00 per year (Canadian institutions), $225.00 per year (Canadian and foreign student/resident), $460.00 per year (foreign individuals), and $830.00 per year (foreign institutions). To receive student and resident rate, orders must be accompanied by name of affiliated institution, date of term, and the *signature* of program/residency coordinator on institutions letterhead. Orders will be billed at individual rate until proof of status is received. Foreign air speed delivery is included in all *Clinics'* subscription prices. All prices are subject to change without notice. POSTMASTER: Send address changes to *Anesthesiology Clinics,* Elsevier Health Sciences Division, Subscription Customer Service, 3251 Riverport Lane, Maryland Heights, MO 63043. Customer Service (orders, claims, online, change of address): Elsevier Health Sciences Division, Subscription Customer Service, 3251 Riverport Lane, Maryland Heights, MO 63043. **Tel:1-800-654-2452 (U.S. and Canada); 314-447-8871 (outside U.S. and Canada). Fax: 314-447-8029. E-mail: journalscustomerservice-usa@elsevier. com (for print support); journalsonlinesupport-usa@elsevier.com (for online support).**

Reprints. For copies of 100 or more of articles in this publication, please contact the Commercial Reprints Department, Elsevier Inc., 360 Park Avenue South, New York, NY 10010-1710. Tel.: 212-633-3874; Fax: 212-633-3820; E-mail: reprints@elsevier.com.

Anesthesiology Clinics, is also published in Spanish by McGraw-Hill Inter-americana Editores S. A., P.O. Box 5-237, 06500 Mexico D. F., Mexico.

Anesthesiology Clinics, is covered in *MEDLINE/PubMed (Index Medicus), Current Contents/Clinical Medicine, Excerpta Medica, ISI/BIOMED*, and *Chemical Abstracts*.

Contributors

CONSULTING EDITOR

LEE A. FLEISHER, MD, FACC, FAHA
Robert D. Dripps Professor and Chair of Anesthesiology and Critical Care, Professor of Medicine, Perelman School of Medicine, University of Pennsylvania, Philadelphia, Pennsylvania

EDITORS

AMR E. ABOULEISH, MD, MBA, FASA
Professor, Department of Anesthesiology, The University of Texas Medical Branch, Galveston, Texas

STANLEY W. STEAD, MD, MBA, FASA
President and CEO, Stead Health Group, Inc, Los Angeles, California

AUTHORS

JOHN ALLYN, MD
Associate Professor, Anesthesiology and Perioperative Medicine, Tufts University School of Medicine, Staff Anesthesiologist, Department of Anesthesiology and Perioperative Medicine, Spectrum Healthcare Partners, Maine Medical Center, Portland, Maine

KEITH J. CHAMBERLIN, MD, MBA
CEO, Chamberlin Health Care Consulting Group, San Rafael, California

CRAIG CURRY, MD
Assistant Professor, Anesthesiology and Perioperative Medicine, Tufts University School of Medicine, Staff Anesthesiologist, Department of Anesthesiology and Perioperative Medicine, Spectrum Healthcare Partners, Maine Medical Center, Portland, Maine

EDWARD J. DAMROSE, MD
Chief of Staff, Stanford Health Care, Associate Professor and Chief, Division of Laryngology, Stanford Health Care, Stanford, California

MARTIN DE RUYTER, MD
Professor, Department of Anesthesiology and Pain Medicine, The University of Kansas Medical Center, Kansas City, Kansas

THOMAS DILLER, MD, MMM
Associate Professor, Department of Health Behavior and Health Systems, School of Public Health, University of North Texas Health Science Center, Executive Director, Institute for Patient Safety, Fort Worth, Texas

MONALIZA GAW, MPA, MSN, CPHQ, NEA-BC, RN
Executive Director of Quality, JPS Health Network, Fort Worth, Texas

MARK E. HUDSON, MD, MBA
Executive Vice Chair, Vice Chair for Clinical Operations, Professor, Department of Anesthesiology, University of Pittsburgh Physicians, University of Pittsburgh School of Medicine, Pittsburgh, Pennsylvania

BASSAM KADRY, MD
Clinical Associate Professor, Anesthesiology, Perioperative, and Pain Medicine, Department of Anesthesiology, Stanford Health Care, Stanford, California

TALAL W. KHAN, MD, MBA
Professor and Chair, Department of Anesthesiology and Pain Medicine, The University of Kansas Medical Center, Kansas City, Kansas

EVAN E. LEBOVITZ, MD
Anesthesiology Resident, CA-2, Department of Anesthesiology, University of Pittsburgh Medical Center, Pittsburgh, Pennsylvania

ALEX MACARIO, MD, MBA
Professor of Anesthesiology, Perioperative and Pain Medicine and, by courtesy, of Health Research and Policy at the Stanford University Medical Center, Department of Anesthesiology, Stanford Health Care, Stanford, California

AMAN MAHAJAN, MD, PhD, MBA
Ronald L. Katz Professor and Chair, Department of Anesthesiology and Perioperative Medicine, UCLA Health, Los Angeles, California

SMITH MANION, MD
Associate Professor, Department of Anesthesiology and Pain Medicine, The University of Kansas Medical Center, Kansas City, Kansas

SHARON K. MERRICK, MS, CCS-P
Director of Payment and Practice Management, American Society of Anesthesiologists, Inc, Washington, DC

AMANDA J. MORRIS, MD
Clinical Instructor, Anesthesiology, Perioperative, and Pain Medicine, Postdoctoral Research Fellow of Management of Perioperative Services, Department of Anesthesiology, Stanford Health Care, Stanford, California

MATTHEW T. POPOVICH, PhD
Director of Quality and Regulatory Affairs, American Society of Anesthesiologists, Washington, DC

JOHN-PAUL J. POZEK, MD
Assistant Professor, Department of Anesthesiology and Pain Medicine, The University of Kansas Medical Center, Kansas City, Kansas

AVIVA REGEV, MD, MBA
Assistant Professor, Department of Anesthesiology and Perioperative Medicine, UCLA Health, Los Angeles, California

FRANK ROSINIA, MD, MHCM
Executive Vice President, Chief Quality Officer, JPS Heath Network, Professor, Department of Health Behavior and Health Systems, School of Public Health, University of North Texas Health Science Center, Fort Worth, Texas

JOSEPH A. SANFORD, MD
Assistant Professor, Anesthesiology, Medical Director, Interventional Services Line, Department of Anesthesiology, University of Arkansas for Medical Sciences, Little Rock, Arkansas

DeLAINE SCHMITZ, MSHL, RN
Quality and Reporting Executive, American Society of Anesthesiologists, Schaumburg, Illinois

MIKE SCHWEITZER, MD, MBA
Principal, Population Health, Premier Inc, Chief Clinical Officer, PSH Learning Collaborative, Clearwater, Florida

NEIL N. SHAH, MD
Assistant Professor, Department of Medicine, Dell Medical School, The University of Texas at Austin, Austin, Texas

STANLEY W. STEAD, MD, MBA, FASA
President and CEO, Stead Health Group, Inc, Los Angeles, California

JOSEPH W. SZOKOL, MD, JD, MBA
Harris Family Foundation Chairman, Department of Anesthesiology, Critical Care and Pain Medicine, NorthShore University HealthSystem, Evanston, Illinois; Clinical Professor, Pritzker School of Medicine, The University of Chicago, Chicago, Illinois

AVERY TUNG, MD, FCCM
Professor, Quality Chief for Anesthesia, Department of Anesthesia and Critical Care, The University of Chicago, Chicago, Illinois

THOMAS R. VETTER, MD, MPH
Professor, Director of Perioperative Care, Departments of Surgery and Perioperative Care and Population Health, Dell Medical School, The University of Texas at Austin, Austin, Texas

SAMUEL H. WALD, MD, MBA
Vice President of Inpatient Perioperative Services, Associate Chief Medical Officer, Perioperative and Interventional Services, Clinical Professor, Department of Anesthesiology, Stanford Health Care, Stanford, California

Contents

Section I: Operating Room Management

Productivity measurements have been used to evaluate and compare physicians and physician practices. Anesthesiology is unique in that factors outside anesthesiologist control affect the opportunity for revenue generation and make comparisons between providers and facilities challenging. This article uses data from the multicenter University of Pittsburgh Physicians Department of Anesthesiology to demonstrate factors influencing productivity opportunity by surgical facility, between department divisions and subspecialties within multispecialty divisions, and by individuals within divisions. The complexities of benchmarking anesthesiology productivity are demonstrated, and the potential value of creating a productivity profile for facilities and groups is illustrated.

A keystone of operating room (OR) management is proper OR allocation to optimize access, safety, efficiency, and throughput. Access is important to surgeons, and overlapping surgery may increase patient access to surgeons with specialized skill sets and facilitate the training of medical students, residents, and fellows. Overlapping surgery is commonly performed in academic medical centers, although recent public scrutiny has raised debate about its safety, necessitating monitoring. This article introduces a system to monitor overlapping surgery, providing a surgeon-specific Key Performance Indicator, and discusses overlapping surgery as an approach toward OR management goals of efficiency and throughput.

Section II: Quality and Reporting

A robust quality management system (QMS) will provide value to patients, providers, and hospitals or systems by focusing on system performance.

The QMS must remain independent of provider-specific measures used for privileging. Some outcome measures may be used to assess system performance; they must not be used to assess individual provider performance. All anesthesia providers, especially leaders, must be guardians of an organization's safety culture.

Although measuring outcomes is an integral part of medical quality improvement, large-scale outcome reporting efforts face several challenges. Among these are difficulties in establishing consensus definitions for outcome measurement; classifying gray outcomes, such as postoperative respiratory failure; and adequately adjusting for patient comorbidities and severity of illness. Unintended consequences of outcome reporting can also distort care in undesirable ways, and clinician reluctance to care for high-risk patients may occur with reporting programs. Ultimately, clinicians need not compare outcomes to improve and should recognize that even outcomes that cannot be precisely quantitated can still be improved.

Since the 1990s, the use of quality measures in health care has grown exponentially. Practices must maintain current knowledge of measures that affect their clinicians locally and understand how assessment of these medical professionals affects the priorities and quality activities of practices and facilities. Because quality measures are increasingly used by hospital administrators, health plans, and payers, practices are being asked to shoulder the additional burdens of collecting and reporting data to various entities. Part of the solution to this increased burden often includes contracting with vendors and outside experts, as well as identifying effective local physician and practice champions.

Since the publication of "To Err is Human" in 1999, substantial efforts have been made within the health care industry to improve quality and patient safety. Although improvements have been made, recent estimates continue to indicate the need for a marked change in approach. In this article, the authors discuss the concepts and characteristics of high reliability organizations, safety culture, and clinical microsystems. The health care delivery system must move beyond current quality and patient safety approaches and fully engage in these new concepts to transform health care system performance.

Section III: Anesthesiology's Value Proposition

Health care in general and anesthesia in particular have seen dramatic changes in the economic landscape. It is vital if anesthesia groups wish to survive and prosper in this new environment to understand the changes occurring in health care and be flexible and proactive in taking on these challenges. More than ever anesthesia groups must be good corporate citizens and seek ways in which to enhance their value to the organization, whether in the operating room or out of operating room locations, and be a proactive partner with the hospital.

treatment of postoperative pain. Physician anesthesiologists have expertise in acute pain management, pharmacology, and regional and neuraxial anesthetic techniques, making them ideal leaders for managing perioperative analgesia within the PSH. Severe postoperative pain is one of many patient- and surgery-specific factors in the development of chronic postsurgical pain. Delivering adequate perioperative analgesia is important to avoid this development, to decrease perioperative morbidity, and to improve patient satisfaction.

In population health medicine, often it is not primary care but rather the specialists' care teams that are responsible for the most overall spending for health care. Engaging specialists in population health medicine is a prerequisite to be successful in improving the quality of care by reducing complications, unnecessary utilization, avoidable emergency department visits/readmissions, and total cost of care. Creating patient-centric, physician-lead, interdisciplinary care teams to redesign the delivery of care across the continuum of the episode of care (eg, shadow bundle) is a successful approach to commercial or Centers for Medicare and Medicaid Services value-based payments.

As health care reform shifts toward value over volume, academic medical centers, known for highly specialized, high-cost care, will suffer from erosion of their traditional funding sources. Academic medical centers have undertaken mergers and partnerships with community medical centers to maintain a more diversified, cost-effective, and competitive presence in their markets. These consolidations have seen varying results. Cultural factors are frequently cited as a cause of dysfunction and disintegration. Anesthesiology groups integrating academic and private practice physicians are likely to face many of the same challenges. Appropriate attention to culture and other key issues may help realize numerous benefits.

ANESTHESIOLOGY CLINICS

THE CLINICS ARE AVAILABLE ONLINE!
Access your subscription at:
www.theclinics.com

Foreword

Practice Management: Successfully Guiding Your Group into the Future

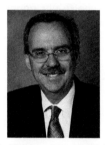

Lee A. Fleisher, MD, FACC, FAHA
Consulting Editor

Medicine is both a noble profession and social good, but is also a business. The future of health care is clearly focused on the value proposition. Within that context, the field of anesthesiology is actively engaged in defining its value. In this issue of the *Anesthesiology Clinics*, the editors have focused on three issues of practice management: operating room management, quality and reporting, and the value proposition. As we attempt to articulate our value to the payers and "employers," such as hospitals, ambulatory surgery centers, and health systems, the information in these articles should prove very useful.

This issue was proposed and edited by two thought-leaders in this arena. Dr Abouleish is a professor of Anesthesiology in the division of pediatric anesthesia at the University of Texas Medical Branch in Galveston, Texas. While at UTMB, he completed his MBA at University of Houston Clear Lake. Dr Abouleish's research interest is the economics of anesthesia care, and specifically, the measurement and benchmarking of clinical productivity in anesthesiologists and anesthesiology groups. He is on several American Society of Anesthesiologists (ASA) committees, including the Committee on Economics and the Committee on Practice Management, for which he is a past chair. Dr Stead is CEO and Founder of the Stead Health Group. He received his MBA from UCLA. He is currently Vice President for Professional Affairs for the ASA. He has extensive experience in health care coding and

Anesthesiology Clin 36 (2018) xiii–xiv
https://doi.org/10.1016/j.anclin.2018.02.003
1932-2275/18/© 2018 Published by Elsevier Inc.

anesthesiology.theclinics.com

payment expertise. Together, they have assembled an amazing group of leaders in our specialty to describe different models of transformation of clinical practice.

Lee A. Fleisher, MD, FACC, FAHA
Perelman School of Medicine
University of Pennsylvania
3400 Spruce Street, Dulles 680
Philadelphia, PA 19104, USA

E-mail address:
Lee.Fleisher@uphs.upenn.edu

Preface

Managing Your Anesthesiology Practice for the Future

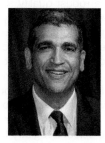   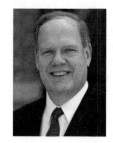

Amr E. Abouleish, MD, MBA, FASA   Stanley W. Stead, MD, MBA, FASA

Editors

Managing your anesthesiology practice for the future continues to be a challenge. In the past, anesthesiology practices focused on volume: maximizing unit production, the conversion factor rate, and account collections. Successful practices minimized their overall costs of billing and administration and carefully managed the number of anesthetizing locations. But health care delivery systems are evolving, and successful anesthesiology groups must expand their traditional focus to meet new demands and challenges. In this issue of *Anesthesiology Clinics*, we present thirteen articles that focus on these new demands and challenges. First, you must be able to measure your production, costs, and quality. Second, anesthesiology practices must expand their comfort zone of the operating room (OR) to include the perioperative period for presurgical optimization, multimodal pain management, and postoperative recovery as exemplified by the perioperative surgical home (PSH). Finally, the traditional divisions of academic and private practice have become blurred to encompass the skills and capabilities of both divisions moving forward.

OPERATING ROOM MANAGEMENT

Even as anesthesiology practices are asked to expand their duties, the primary challenge of surgical anesthesia continues. But unlike previous years, many anesthesiology groups do not simply cover one facility but now are part of large groups or national companies that cover multiple facilities. With this expansion of coverage, groups are trying to make data-driven evaluations on productivity and OR efficiencies. Hudson and Lebovitz present their lessons learned from comparing clinical productivity among 14 different facilities. Morris and colleagues describe principles of OR efficiency and how they apply to a real-world scenario: one surgeon wanting to "flip"

Anesthesiology Clin 36 (2018) xv–xvii
https://doi.org/10.1016/j.anclin.2018.02.002
1932-2275/18/© 2018 Published by Elsevier Inc.

anesthesiology.theclinics.com

cases in two rooms. Methods and measures are described for monitoring overlapping surgery, auditing, providing accountability and metrics of surgical production.

QUALITY AND REPORTING

Quality outcome reporting has become an important requirement of many practices, not only to federal payers but also to the practice, facilities, and other payers. Focusing on individual clinicians, Allyn and Curry describe a robust quality system based upon the data collected from their department that has evolved over 20 years. They describe how to capture data, how to provide meaningful reporting of the information, and how to use that data to demonstrate the value their practice brings to their institution. Tung reminds the reader of the challenges of outcome reporting: avoiding direct comparisons between clinicians, while still providing a framework for institutional improvement of outcome reporting. In contrast to Allyn and Curry, Popovich and Schmitz focus on group quality reporting. They discuss measure development and how those measures are captured into clinical data registries. They provide readers with a wealth of information on reporting and how to select a registry for reporting quality outcome measures. Facilities are also very interested in developing quality organizations. Rosinia and colleagues expand the concepts of quality reporting and safety into principles for anesthesiology's development of a high-reliability organization in intensive care and ORs.

ANESTHESIOLOGY'S VALUE PROPOSITION

Anesthesiology practices must continue to evolve and articulate measurable and demonstrable benefits that patients, facilities, other providers, and payers receive from an anesthesia service. Practices must be able to compete by moving from piecework to bundled payments. Those bundles must encompass the continuum of care from the decision to operate to recovery of function. Termed the PSH, practices must optimize the patient for surgery, manage their recovery and pain management, and encompass population health. Szokol and Chamberlin analyze the strengths, weaknesses, and opportunities practices face. They conclude with recommendations that practice must seize: leadership, patient satisfaction, and incorporation of the PSH into their practice. Stead and Merrick take readers through the considerations and analysis of the services and costs of providing anesthesia services for an episode of care. They show the calculations and decisions necessary to develop a bundled payment for all anesthesia services needed during an episode of surgical care.

Anesthesiology's expanded role in preoperative assessment and preparation for surgery is highlighted by Shah and Vetter. They articulate the use of graded assessments from mobile technologies to face-to-face visits to assess comorbidities, optimize patients, and provide prehabilitation with targeted therapeutic interventions. Principles of PSH can also be applied to pain medicine. Pozek and colleagues illustrate how improved and coordinated acute pain management of surgical patients can have even more impact than simply shortened length of stay. Careful preoperative assessment of risk factors, including behavioral risk factors, perioperative management with multimodal nonopioid analgesia, and regional and neuraxial techniques, can minimize postsurgical pain and minimize the risk of chronic postsurgical pain. Khan and Manion describe how the PSH can provide an optimal framework for complex chronic pain patients. Chronic pain patients benefit from preoperative assessment with optimization in planning for surgery, with the use of intraoperative multimodal analgesia. Postoperative and postdischarge care coordination care pathways in the PSH are essential for chronic pain patients.

Schweitzer believes that expansion beyond the PSH to engaging anesthesiologists and the surgical specialists in population health will improve quality, reduce costs, and provide more effective care management processes. He encourages anesthesiologists to participate in accountable care organizations and population health management organizations to develop "shadow bundles" to improve quality and reduce costs.

In the final article, Regev and Mahajan describe the opportunities and challenges in merging academic and private practice anesthesiology groups. These mergers are often done to gain efficiencies and synergies, but the differences between these two types of practices in their workforces and workflow can affect the overall success of a merger.

Amr E. Abouleish, MD, MBA, FASA
Department of Anesthesiology
The University of Texas Medical Branch
301 University Boulevard
Galveston, TX 77555-0877, USA

Stanley W. Stead, MD, MBA, FASA
Stead Health Group, Inc
4819 Andasol Avenue, Suite 100
Encino, CA 91316-3802, USA

E-mail addresses:
aaboulei@utmb.edu (A.E. Abouleish)
sstead@gmail.com (S.W. Stead)

Section I: Operating Room Management

Measuring Clinical Productivity

Mark E. Hudson, MD, MBA[a],*, Evan E. Lebovitz, MD[b]

KEYWORDS

- Benchmarking • Clinical performance • Clinical productivity • Clinical efficiency
- Practice management • Anesthesiology • ASA unit production

KEY POINTS

- Evaluation of clinical productivity and comparison of providers and facilities is uniquely challenging in anesthesiology because various factors outside anesthesiologist control impact opportunity for revenue generation.
- An understanding of the factors impacting productivity in anesthesiology can allow for adjustments in fair workload and compensation distribution within performance-based compensation plans or with productivity incentives.
- Although total ASA units (tASA) per FTE is the primary productivity metric, numerous factors influence opportunity for tASA generation, such as concurrency, OR use, call burden, case type and length, OR scheduling and case management, and non-ASA generating essential duties.
- Creating an anesthesiology productivity profile for facilities and groups can allow for better evaluation and comparison of productivity within an institution or with existing national data.

INTRODUCTION

Measuring and comparing clinical productivity in the practice of anesthesiology is complex, because benchmarking work between facilities and individuals outside of a group or company must be done with the limited information that exists with available practice survey data. To effectively evaluate effort and efficiency of work and have meaningful comparisons between individuals and groups, opportunity differences in productivity need to be fully understood and appreciated. These opportunity differences occur between facilities, groups or divisions, subspecialties within a

Disclosure Statement: N/A.
[a] Department of Anesthesiology, University of Pittsburgh Physicians, University of Pittsburgh School of Medicine, Suite A-1305, Scaife Hall, 3550 Terrace Street, Pittsburgh, PA 15262, USA;
[b] Department of Anesthesiology, University of Pittsburgh Medical Center, Kaufman Medical Building, Suite 910, 3471 Fifth Avenue, Pittsburgh, PA 15213, USA
* Corresponding author.
E-mail address: hudsonme@anes.upmc.edu

Anesthesiology Clin 36 (2018) 143–160
https://doi.org/10.1016/j.anclin.2018.01.001
1932-2275/18/© 2018 Elsevier Inc. All rights reserved.
anesthesiology.theclinics.com

group, and individuals. In this article, we present the results of our department's detailed process and lessons learned in the measurement and comparison of clinical productivity of nine department divisions accounting for coverage of 14 distinct facilities by more than 140 clinical anesthesiology physician full-time equivalents (FTE). Through demonstrating our process and in-depth understanding, the goal is to give the reader the tools to understand how to measure clinical productivity and describe the factors that affect these variables, the process for making more meaningful comparisons between divisions and individuals within a group or company, and the ability to monitor factors impacting productivity to allow for data-driven planning and goal setting.

Productivity measurements have long been used to evaluate and compare physicians and physician practices because many practices use these data to develop incentives or performance-based compensation plans.[1] In this respect, work relative value units have been considered the gold standard to measure physician productivity, in part because they have a basis in the resource-based relative value scale method, an approach reflecting the relative level of time, skill, stress, and education necessary to perform a given task. Work relative value units, therefore, allow for the calculation of the volume of work and effort expended by a physician and are used to compare physicians within a given specialty. Anesthesiology, however, uses a more complex approach based on a different relative value system, the American Society of Anesthesiologists (ASA) Relative Value Guide, which measures work based on three components that sum to total ASA units (tASA) per case: (1) a base unit reflecting the complexity of the preoperative evaluation and difficulty of planning and performing the anesthetic, (2) time units that reflect the total time engaged in the care of the patient, and (3) modifier units.

The difference between these two methodologies was successfully lobbied for with the introduction of the resource-based relative value scale method because of the demonstrated impact on revenue/expense by factors unassociated with individual effort, primarily variance in surgical case time for a given procedure.[2] Even with this anesthesiology-specific methodology, case type and length differences impact opportunity for tASA production.[3,4] Furthermore, other influencing factors beyond group or individual practitioner control contribute to opportunity differences for tASA unit generation making comparisons between providers particularly challenging.[5]

The current health care economic environment has led to an increased interest in productivity and efficiency as hospitals seek to improve fiscal viability through efforts aimed at reducing costs of care delivery. Benchmarking anesthesiology productivity is increasingly being used by hospitals and health care organizations to assess the value of anesthesiology expenses, and is frequently included as a contractual condition within groups or for individual providers. Although external anesthesiology productivity benchmarking data are available from organizations, such as the Medical Group Management Association and the American Medical Group Association, these tools are largely incomplete and insufficient to effectively compare practices or individual providers. This is largely caused by the broad and varied differences in factors within practices whose impact on productivity is not fully understood or accounted for in survey-based data collection approaches. These shortcomings have led to efforts in understanding and adjusting for practice variables to allow clinical productivity comparisons and articulate specific practice conditions impacting anesthesiologist productivity.[3–8] An understanding of these factors can allow adjustments to be made for fair workload and compensation distribution within performance-based compensation plans or productivity incentive programs.

GENERATION OF AMERICAN SOCIETY OF ANESTHESIOLOGISTS UNITS PER FULL-TIME EQUIVALENTS

The primary productivity metric used for anesthesiologists is tASA per clinical FTE (tASA/FTE). **Fig. 1** demonstrates how tASA/FTE is generated with illustrations of key factors influencing productivity. Each case is associated with base unit and time unit generation, which sum to tASA/case with the total cases per hour available creating the tASA per billable hour opportunity. Operating room (OR) and case management efficiency along with concurrency (CONC) determine how this opportunity per billable hour translates into tASA per work hour for individual anesthesiologists. tASA per work hour generation is maximized during surgical "prime time" when CONC, OR use, and efficiency are at their peak. Second shift and call burden, which are associated with a reduction in opportunity for tASA/h generation per anesthesiologist, reduces the tASA per work hour. The work hours associated with non-ASA unit generation further dilute the tASA per work hour. The total work hours necessary for an FTE then determines the tASA/FTE. This figure demonstrates the multiple variables likely to influence tASA/FTE generation, many of which are outside anesthesiologist control, including case type and length of surgery, OR scheduling and case management, efficiency, non-ASA generating essential duties, and required call coverage.

ASSESSMENT OF DEPARTMENTAL PRODUCTIVITY

Data collection encompassed a full fiscal year of billing, clinical activity, and surgical services data for the University of Pittsburgh Physicians Department of Anesthesiology across nine separate divisions covering 14 total individual surgical facilities, including total base units and time units generated per faculty by facility and division, scheduling data, and clinical FTE per faculty by division. Patient anonymity in data collections was strictly maintained via deidentification by the administrative team.

We compared clinical productivity metrics by surgical facility, between department divisions, by subspecialties within complex multispecialty divisions, and by individual anesthesiologists within divisions. Furthermore, we evaluated the factors thought to impact productivity opportunities and demonstrate the complexities of benchmarking

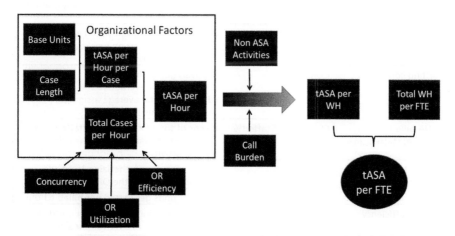

Fig. 1. Generation of tASA/FTE with key factors influencing productivity. OR, operating room; WH, work hours. (*From* Hudson ME. Benchmarking anesthesiologists' performance: understanding factors that impact productivity. ASA Monitor 2016;80:41; with permission.)

anesthesiologist productivity. Additionally, we illustrate the potential value of creating a productivity profile for facilities and groups allowing comparison of factors influencing productivity. **Table 1** provides a summary of data collected, variables, and definitions used throughout this report.

The nine separate divisions studied are listed in **Table 2**. The divisions are rank ordered by size based on clinical FTE with documentation of key characteristics

Table 1 Data collected, variables, and definitions		
Measure	**Abbreviation**	**Definition and Comments**
Base units billed	B	For one full fiscal year, July 1–June 30, including all activity billed via ASA RVG methodology
Time units billed	TU	For one full fiscal year, July 1–June 30, including all activity billed via ASA RVG methodology
Total ASA units billed	tASA	For one full fiscal year, July 1–June 30, including all activity billed via ASA RVG methodology
Billable hours	h	Equals TU divided by 4; one time unit equals 15 min
Total cases performed	Case	For one full fiscal year, July 1–June 30, including all activity billed via ASA RVG methodology
Average number of anesthetizing sites staffed daily	OR	For one full fiscal year, July 1–June 30, including all non-OR anesthetizing locations
Clinical FTEs	FTE	Total full time equivalents for full fiscal year associated with clinical anesthesiology care delivery, including call; one FTE = 230 Shift Equivalents
Clinical day	d	Total weekdays exclusive of holidays for full fiscal year = 252
Percent of FTE associated with call	CallFTE%	Percent of total FTE associated with care provided after 7 PM on weekdays and 24 h on weekend days
Staffing concurrency	CONC	7 AM average staffing staffing concurrency = average rooms staffed divided by total average assigned anesthesiologists
CRNA billed time per clinical staffed time	CRNABilled/Staffed%	Percent of total CRNA clinical staffed time that is associated with anesthesiology billing activity
Percent NORA Locations	NORA %	Percent of total anesthetizing locations located outside of the ORs
Billable hour efficiency	tASA/h	Total ASA units generated per billable hour
Staffing efficiency	OR/FTE	Total anesthetizing locations per day divided by total clinical FTE for full fiscal year

Includes definitions and abbreviations of collected data and key terms as they apply throughout the analysis.
Abbreviations: ASA RVG, ASA Relative Value Guide; CRNA, certified registered nurse anesthetist.

Table 2
Division composition and key staffing elements

	Adult/PED	FTE	ORs	NORA	TotalLoc	NORA%	Teaching	IHCall	BpCall	CallFTE%	CONC	CRNABilled/Staffed%
Division I												
QUAT	Adult	—	36	13	49	—	—	—	—	—	—	—
Total	—	34	36	13	49	27	Yes	1	2	15	2.1	61.0
Division II												
QPED	Peds	—	14	5	—	—	—	—	—	—	—	—
ASC	Peds	—	4	0	—	—	—	—	—	—	—	—
Total	—	24	18	5	23	22	Yes	1	2	13	1.4	63.0
Division III												
TERT	Adult	—	23	3	26	—	—	—	—	—	—	—
ASC	Adult	—	2.5	0	2.5	—	—	—	—	—	—	—
Total	—	20	25.5	3	28.5	11	No	1	1	18	2.2	60.0
Division IV												
TERT	Adult	—	18	5	24	—	—	—	—	—	—	—
Total	—	17	18	5	24	21	Yes	2	2	38	2.4	58.0
Division V												
COM	Adult	—	16	5	21	—	—	—	—	—	—	—
ASC	Adult	—	5	0	5	—	—	—	—	—	—	—
Total	—	15	21	5	26	19	No	0	2	12	2.6	65.0

(continued on next page)

Table 2
(continued)

	Adult/PED	FTE	ORs	NORA	TotalLoc	NORA%	Teaching	IHCall	BpCall	CallFTE%	CONC	CRNABilled/Staffed%
Division VI												
COM	Adult	—	15	1	16	—	—	—	—	—	—	—
Total	—	13	15	1	16	6	No	1	1	7	2.7	65.0
Division VII												
COM	Adult	—	14	0	14	—	—	—	—	—	—	—
ASC	Adult	—	5	0	5	—	—	—	—	—	—	—
Total	—	10	19	0	19	0	No	0	1	13	2.7	64.0
Division VIII												
COM	Adult	—	5	1	6	—	—	—	—	—	—	—
COM	Adult	—	4	1	5	—	—	—	—	—	—	—
Total	—	8	9	2	11	18	No	0	1	16	2.2	47.0
Division IX												
COM	Adult	—	3	1	4	—	—	—	—	—	—	—
Total	—	3.5	3	1	4	25	No	0	1	32	2	45.0

Divisions are rank ordered by size based on clinical FTE. Call is defined as coverage between 7 PM and 7 AM, Monday through Friday plus weekends including in-house coverage and pager call (CallFTE%). Facility type is categorized as ambulatory surgical center (ASC), community hospital (COM), tertiary care facility (TERT), pediatric quaternary care facility (QPED), or adult quaternary care facility (QUAT).

Abbreviations: BpCall, beeper call; IHCall, in-house call; TotalLoc, total anesthetizing locations.

including the ORs, non-OR anesthetizing locations (NORA), total anesthetizing locations covered, average 7 AM staffing ratio (CONC), call requirements including in-house call and beeper call, and percentage of total FTE associated with call defined as coverage between 7 PM and 7 AM and Monday through Friday plus weekends including in-house coverage and pager call (CallFTE%). Facility type is categorized as ambulatory surgical center (ASC), community hospital (COM), tertiary care facility (TERT), quaternary care facility (QUAT), or pediatric quaternary facility (QPED). We also included measures of OR and provider use in our analysis. In our health system, CRNA billed time per clinical time worked (CRNABilled/Staffed%) is used as our primary measure of OR efficiency,[9] and this percentage is indicated for each division. Additionally, because of constraints in use and efficiency of NORA, the percentage of NORA locations of total anesthetizing locations is included for each division (NORA%).

A medical direction model of care delivery is used by all sites and a standard demand schedule methodology was used to calculate staffing needs. The definition of a clinical FTE is standard between divisions defined as 230 clinical shift-equivalents per year. In-house call and beeper call shift equivalency calculations were also standard between divisions. All activities generating ASA units were included in the analysis, including obstetric anesthesia services. Dedicated FTEs in the department associated with non-ASA unit generating clinical activity were excluded from the analysis, including those involved in chronic pain, acute pain, and critical care medicine.

Organizational (Facility-Based) Productivity and Benchmarking

Opportunities for tASA generation depend on total available case volume, organizational factors influencing case length and complexity, and distribution of these cases within various anesthetizing locations. Abouleish and colleagues[3,4] demonstrated how these differences can influence tASA opportunity. To develop productivity metrics not impacted by staffing ratios and create meaningful comparisons of anesthesiology practices, their group developed productivity metrics based on per anesthetizing location and per case measures, demonstrating differences by facility type and size, type of surgical staff, and academic versus private practice. In their study, they found that ASCs had significantly lower tASA per OR site (tASA/OR), fewer billable hours per OR per day (h/OR/d), and fewer billable hours per case (h/case) than non-ASC hospitals. COM had significantly fewer h/OR/d and h/case than academic medical centers and indigent hospitals. Academic hospitals had significantly lower tASA per hour (tASA/h) and greater h/case.[4] Although differences exist between type of hospital, no two hospitals are exactly alike in these metrics and opportunity for tASA production always varies. However, this methodology does allow the inclusion of a case type and scheduling profile to identify differences in opportunity for production by facility or within groups, and provides more valid benchmarks by facility type.

Applying this methodology to our data set, we evaluated differences and trends in our covered surgical facilities and identified organizational factors that may impact productivity opportunity. Facilities were categorized as Ambulatory Surgical Center (ASC); COM defined as a hospital without a full complement of adult subspecialty surgical care delivery; TERT defined as a hospital providing a full complement of adult subspecialty care; an adult QUAT providing a full complement of complex subspecialty care, trauma, and transplantation; and a QPED providing a full complement of complex pediatric surgeries including transplantation. **Table 3** shows productivity by covered facility on a per case and per OR basis including total cases and start of day average anesthetizing sites (ORs), with calculated tASA per OR (tASA/OR), billable hours (time units divided by four) per case (h/case), tASA per billable hour (tASA/h),

Table 3
Facility productivity per case and per operating room

	Cases	ORs	tASA/OR	h/OR/d	h/Case	tASA/h	Base/h	Base/ Case	tASA/ Case	tASA/ OR/d
ASC	7591	3.5	16,455	6.47	0.76	10.04	6.04	4.57	7.59	65.3
	8764	5	13,863	5.99	0.86	9.15	5.15	4.45	7.91	55.0
	5825	3	17,438	8.46	1.10	8.15	4.15	4.57	8.98	69.2
	2902	2.6	9952	5.19	1.18	7.58	3.58	4.21	8.92	39.5
Total	25,082	14.1	14,546	6.53	0.92	8.86	4.86	4.49	8.18	57.7
COM	7703	6	13,628	7.06	1.39	7.63	3.63	5.05	10.62	54.1
	21,535	21	13,152	6.97	1.72	7.46	3.46	5.95	12.83	52.2
	26,712	16	19,122	10.19	1.54	7.42	3.42	5.28	11.45	75.9
	5521	5	10,869	5.87	1.34	7.32	3.32	4.47	9.84	43.1
	13,497	14	12,161	6.62	1.74	7.26	3.26	5.66	12.61	48.3
	4740	4	12,865	7.03	1.50	7.24	3.24	4.86	10.86	51.1
Total	79,708	66	14,242	7.63	1.59	7.40	3.40	5.42	11.79	56.5
QPED	20,615	19	14,532	8.14	1.90	7.06	3.06	5.80	13.39	57.7
TERT	20,438	24	11,239	6.35	1.89	7.00	3.00	5.65	13.20	44.6
	20,762	26	12,791	7.36	2.33	6.87	2.87	6.69	16.02	50.8
Total	41,200	50	12,046	6.90	2.11	6.93	2.93	6.18	14.62	47.8
QUAT	36,477	49	13,062	8.02	2.73	6.44	2.44	6.64	17.55	51.8

Listed for each facility type are productivity on a per case and per OR basis including total cases and start of day average anesthetizing sites (ORs), with calculated tASA per OR (tASA/OR), billable hours (time units divided by four) per case (h/case), tASA per billable hour (tASA/h), base units per billable hour (base/h), base units per case (base/case), tASA per case (tASA/case), billable hours per OR per day (h/OR/d), and tASA per OR per day (tASA/OR/d).

base units per billable hour (base/h), base units per case (base/case), tASA per case (tASA/case), billable hours per OR per day (h/OR/d), and tASA per OR per day (tASA/OR/d).

In comparing these productivity metrics by type of facility, we found no difference in tASA/OR among ASCs, COM, or QPED facilities; however, we discovered lower tASA/OR for our TERT and QUAT facilities. h/case and tASA/case increased with increasing complexity of facility from ASC to QUAT with tASA/h highest in our ASCs and trending downward through our QUAT facility. **Fig. 2** shows the tASA/h by individual facility and facility type and the h/case for each facility. ASCs generated the highest tASA/h followed by COM, QPED, TERT, and QUAT facilities. tASA/h correlates strongly negatively ($r = -0.84$) with anesthetic duration (hours billed per case). h/case correlates strongly positively with tASA/case ($r = 0.92$). There was little difference in average tASA/OR/d between our ASCs, COM, and QPED sites, with lower tASA/OR/d found in our TERT and QUAT sites.

This information allows for the development of a profile for each facility and for a comparison of case type and length, anesthetizing locations, and potential differences in productivity opportunity by facility. With staffing typically based on total anesthetizing location coverage needed, tASA/OR/d is the metric most likely to influence tASA opportunity per FTE, and a review of sites with low tASA/OR/d illuminates this primary constraint. For example, within our ASCs, one facility lags considerably in tASA/OR/d. In this facility, the case length (h/case) is higher than expected for the average base unit per case, suggesting a longer average case length for the complexity of cases performed. Additionally, this site has the lowest h/OR/d of our ASC sites. Within our community sites, one facility also trails the others in tASA/OR/d. At this

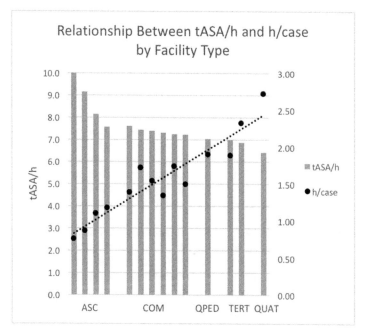

Fig. 2. tASA per FTE by individual facility and facility type and h/case for each facility. ASCs generated the highest tASA per billed hours (tASA/h) followed by COM, QPED, TERT, and QUAT facilities. tASA/h correlated strongly negatively (r = −0.84) with anesthetic duration (h/case).

site, h/OR/d is the lowest of the group. The facility in the COM group with the highest tASA/OR/d has the highest h/OR/d of any of our facilities.

Group (Division) Productivity and Benchmarking

Although measuring productivity by facility on a per OR and per case approach provides important insight into the factors impacting opportunity for tASA generation, it is important to recognize that these factors alone may not correlate with overall division or individual productivity per FTE, in part because of other influencing factors relating to generation of tASA units per FTE (see **Fig. 1**). A per OR and per case approach only provides the available opportunity based on tASA units per billable hour, which represents the time that a provider is associated with the case. Therefore, it does not necessarily represent the overall opportunity on a per work hour basis. Anesthetizing location efficiency and use, work hours associated with non-ASA unit generation for clinical faculty, and CONC all affect tASA unit production per work hour and ultimately per FTE. Furthermore, it is important to account for non-primetime periods and call activities, which are intrinsically associated with a reduced opportunity for tASA unit generation. These OR and staffing efficiencies vary by facility and within groups, adding to the difficulty in making meaningful comparisons.

To evaluate potential factors impacting group productivity, we proceeded in a complex analysis of organizational factors by division (tASA/h, h/OR/d, h/case, base/case, tASA/h, tASA/case), staffing efficiencies (CONC and % of total FTE associated with call), and OR efficiency. We used our previously described CRNA billed time to staffed time (CRNABilled/Staffed%) as our measure of OR efficiency.[9] With the growth of

NORA and the associated decreased use and efficiency,[10,11] percent of NORA locations to total locations (%NORA) was included in the analysis. **Table 4** illustrates the results of the analysis for each of the nine divisions responsible for the coverage of the 14 surgical facilities.

Distribution of individual productivity within each division was compared on a per FTE basis with significant differences found in tASA/FTE between divisions. Further evaluation was performed comparing tASA/FTE with each of the listed variables to establish possible correlation. **Fig. 3** shows the correlation and r value associated with each variable. tASA/FTE had a strong positive correlation with billable hours per FTE (h/FTE; $P<.01$) and CONC ($P<.01$), and had a high positive correlation with CRNA billed to staffed hours percent (CRNA h/staffed h), although this did not reach statistical significance. tASA/FTE was negatively correlated with call FTE percent (CallFTE%; $P<.05$) and NORA%. A moderate degree of positive correlation was found between tASA/FTE and tASA/OR, h/OR/d, and tASA/h, although these did not reach statistical significance.

The three divisions with tASA/FTE greater than 23,000 (Divisions V, VI, and VII) are all top three performers in billable hours per FTE, 7 AM staffing ratio, CRNA billed to staffed percent, and have the lowest three values for call FTE percent. Review of the three divisions with tASA/FTE less than 15,000 showed that one (Division II, our pediatric division) is distinguished by its low staffing ratio (CONC = 1.4). The other two (Divisions IV and IX) were distinguished by their high CallFTE%.

Individual Productivity and Benchmarking

Productivity opportunities differ between facilities and between groups. Because it is difficult if not impossible to develop a scheduling system to allow equal opportunity for tASA generation for each provider, taking into consideration differences in opportunity based on assignments or call loads may help develop more accurate comparisons of productivity based on individual effort.

Fig. 4 shows the tASA/FTE by site, grouped by size from large (>20 FTE), to medium (10–20 FTE), to small (<10 FTE). University of Pittsburgh Physicians Department of Anesthesiology individual department tASA per clinical FTE distribution is shown using box plots. Interquartile ranges (IQRs) tended to be broadest in sites with subspecialty groups or those covering multiple facilities suggesting the potential impact of assignment or staffing efficiency per subspecialty in large, complex (multispecialty) sites or differences in opportunity if assigned preferentially to multifacility divisions. Small, noncomplex sites had the narrowest IQRs.

To further evaluate tASA/FTE by subspecialty, we compared tASA/FTE productivity by subspecialty type within Division I, our largest and most complex site (**Fig. 5**). Significant differences in tASA/FTE were found between the neuroanesthesiology group, the cardiac, and the transplantation anesthesiology groups ($P<.0001$). Cardiac and transplant subspecialties had a higher call burden, lower CONC, and lower tASA/h than the neuroanesthesiology group.

Reviewing outlier anesthesiologists in tASA/FTE (data points >1.5 times the IQR) revealed that all had differential assignments either by surgical facility or specific case type assignments within a single facility. For example, Division I had one notable outlier, generating 44,143 tASA/FTE compared with a division mean of 19,589. This anesthesiologist was assigned only to the gastrointestinal laboratory daily and did not participate in late or call shifts. Division II, responsible for coverage of a pediatric ASC and a QPED, also had one outlier, generating 23,748 tASA/FTE, compared with a division mean of 14,559. Billing activity demonstrated preferential daily assignment to the ASC for this individual. Compared with the QPED, the pediatric ASC has a higher

Table 4
Organizational, staffing, and efficiency factors by division

Division	FTE	ORs	Cases	tASA/FTE	h/FTE	tASA/OR	h/OR/d	h/Case	tASA/h	tASA/Case	CallFTE%	CONC	CRNABilled/Staffed%
I	34	49	36,477	18,825	2924	13,062.1	8.1	2.7	6.4	17.5	15%	2.1	61
II	24	22.5	28,206	13,904	1869	14,831.2	7.9	1.6	7.4	11.8	13%	1.4	63
III	20	26	20,762	16,628	2420	12,790.9	7.4	2.3	6.9	16.0	18%	2.2	60
IV	17	24	20,438	13,582	1957	9620.6	5.5	1.6	6.9	11.3	38%	2.4	58
V	14	24	27,360	23,464	3103	13,687.5	7.2	1.6	7.6	12.0	12%	2.6	65
VI	13	16	26,712	23,535	3173	19,122.3	10.2	1.5	7.4	11.5	7%	2.7	65
VII	10	19	22,261	23,957	3104	12,608.8	6.5	1.4	7.7	10.8	13%	2.7	64
VIII	8	11	13,224	17,014	2268	12,373.9	6.5	1.4	7.5	10.3	16%	2.2	47
IX	3.5	4	4740	14,703	2032	12,865.0	7.1	1.5	7.2	10.9	32%	2.0	45

Organizational factors by division (tASA/FTE, h/FTE, tASA/OR, h/OR/d, h/case, tASA/h, tASA/case), staffing efficiencies (CallFTE% and CONC), and OR efficiency (CRNABilled/Staffed%) are displayed. Results are shown for each of the nine divisions responsible for the coverage of the 14 surgical facilities.

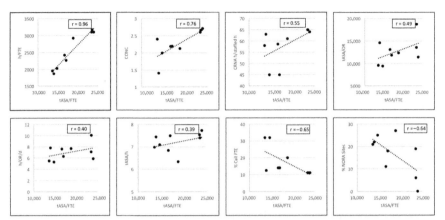

Fig. 3. tASA/FTE correlated with factors impacting productivity. tASA/FTE had a strong positive correlation with billable hours per FTE (h/FTE; $P<.01$), and a strong positive correlation with CONC ($P<.01$), and CRNA billed to staffed hours' percent (CRNA h/staffed h). tASA/FTE was negatively correlated with CallFTE% ($P<.05$) and NORA%. A moderate degree of positive correlation was found between tASA/FTE and tASA/OR, h/OR/d, and tASA/h.

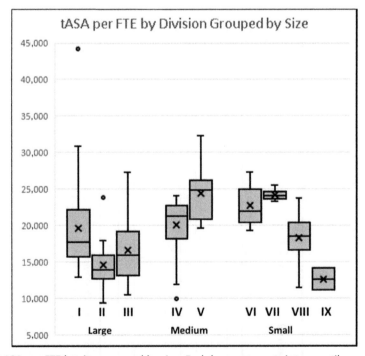

Fig. 4. tASA per FTE by site, grouped by size. Each box represents interquartile range (IQR) divided by a line representing the median. X is the mean; the whiskers extend to a maximum of 1.5 times the IQR beyond the box. Open circles represent data point outliers and are described in the text.

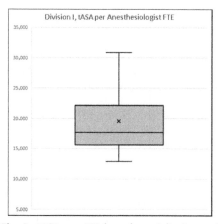 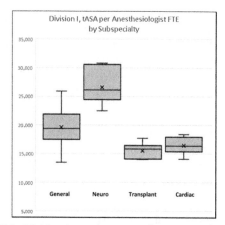

Fig. 5. tASA per FTE by subspecialty type within Division I, our largest and most complex site. Significant differences in tASA/FTE were found between the neuroanesthesiology group (neuro) and the cardiac (cardiac) and transplantation (transplant) anesthesiology groups (*P*<.0001).

tASA/OR/d (65 vs 57) and a higher average staffing ratio (1.75 vs 1.14) affording additional opportunities for tASA generation per shift.

Statistical Methods

Comparison of continuous values among hospital sites or subspecialty was performed using Kruskal-Wallis test with post hoc test using the Dunn multiple comparison method for the data with nonparametric distribution. The level of significance was set at *P* value less than .05. Statistical analysis was performed using GraphPad Prism 7 (GraphPad Software, Inc, La Jolla, CA). Pearson correlation coefficients were computed between tASA/FTE and factors suspected of impacting productivity and data were analyzed using IBM (International Business Machines Corp, Armonk, NY) SPSS Statistics version 22. The level of significance was set at *P* value of less than .05. Because the analysis work was considered exploratory and meant to generate hypotheses for future work, it was not adjusted for multiple comparisons.

DISCUSSION

The standard physician productivity metric of tASA unit production per FTE is not a direct reflection of anesthesiologist work effort. Our data illustrate that even within a single multihospital practice using a standard care team model, standard calculation of FTE need, and standard expected work per FTE, a wide variance in productivity per FTE exists between sites, divisions, and between individuals within divisions. This is a result of the wide-ranging and numerous factors that impact the opportunity for productivity within anesthesiology practices. To make meaningful comparisons between groups or individuals based on effort, an understanding of factors beyond the control of an individual anesthesiologist is required. It is helpful to categorize these factors into billable hour efficiency/organizational factors, anesthesiology staffing efficiency, anesthetizing location efficiency, and non-ASA generating activities.

Billable Hour Efficiency/Organizational Factors

Billable hour efficiency, as defined as tASA units generated per billable hour, indicates the impact of base units and case length on tASA unit production. Base units reflect case complexity of preoperative evaluation, case planning, and performance of the anesthetic. Case length for a given surgical procedure can vary significantly by surgeon or site and is determined by surgeon, facility-specific proficiency, and presence of trainees. Our study confirms the conclusions of those previously published, that billable hour efficiency is highest with short duration cases and declines with increasing case times[3–6] (see **Fig. 2**).

Billable hour efficiency represents the foundation for tASA productivity per FTE. Within the sites covered by our group, it accounts for differences in opportunity for tASA/FTE. As an example, Division II, our pediatric specialty group, covers a pediatric ASC with a billable hour efficiency of 10 tASA/h and a QPED with a billable hour efficiency of 7, representing a 43% increased opportunity for tASA unit production per billable hour at the ASC as compared with the main hospital.

Staffing Efficiency

Our data indicate that staffing efficiency, defined as the number of anesthetizing locations per total clinical FTE, is impacted by CONC, work hours, and percent of total FTE associated with activity after 7 PM on weekdays and all day on weekends (CallFTE%). Staffing efficiency ranges from 0.9 to 1.9. Staffing ratio (CONC), defined as average start of the day anesthetizing sites per assigned anesthesiologist, ranges from 1.2 to 2.7 between divisions. CallFTE% ranges from a low of 7% to a high of 38% of total FTE. Staffing ratio or CONC is primarily limited by case type and complexity, presence of trainees, and facility factors impacting the total sites running, including the geography of those sites. In our analysis, the division with the lowest staffing efficiency (Division II) has the highest number of trainees (residents, fellows, and SRNAs) assigned daily. Accreditation Council for Graduate Medical Education (ACGME) limitations, CMS teaching rules for resident physicians, and the CMS CONC limitations for SRNAs, and case complexity at the QPED further impact CONC at this site. Division IV staffing efficiency is primarily limited by CallFTE%. This site of modest size (17 total FTE) has a call burden of 38%, which is associated with OB coverage, trauma coverage, and the need for pediatric and cardiac anesthesiology subspecialty coverage. Per shift equivalent tASA productivity during call shifts averages 17% of that during noncall shifts within this facility.

Operating Room/Anesthetizing Location Efficiency

Organizational factors affecting anesthesiologist productivity include available surgical hours per staffed anesthetizing location and case volume management efficiency. Prolonged turnovers and excessive gaps between cases reduce tASA per work hour and therefore tASA/FTE. Geography of sites and total rooms running can also limit the optimal CONC. Efficient use of anesthesiology personnel falls dramatically after prime-time hours as efficient case management declines and the number of sites falls below a level allowing optimal CONC. Furthermore, over the past decade, NORA demands have grown contributing to concurrent issues in operational efficiency. Previous studies have highlighted the low utilization rates and the divergence in physician and scheduling efficiency in NORA environments.[10,11] In our review, NORA% seems to be an influencing factor in tASA/FTE.

Non–American Society of Anesthesiologists Generating Activities

Non-ASA generating activities also dilute the tASA/FTE. As practices add activities that do not directly contribute to generation of tASA, tASA/FTE declines. These duties are associated with limited to no additional value for the group or health care organization (increased regulatory or administrative burden) or add significant value in overall care delivery (enhanced recovery after surgery [ERAS] or perioperative surgical home

Table 5
Productivity profile by division

Division	Billable Hour Efficiency/Organizational Factors						Staffing Efficiency			OR Efficiency	
	tASA/FTE	h/Case	tASA/h	tASA/Case	h/OR/d	tASA/OR/d	OR/FTE	CONC	CallFTE%	CRNABilled/Staffed%	NORA%
I	18,825	2.7	6.4	17.5	8.1	51.8	1.4	2.1	15	61	27
II	13,904	1.6	7.4	11.8	7.9	58.9	0.9	1.4	13	63	22
III	16,628	2.3	6.9	16.0	7.4	50.8	1.4	2.2	18	60	11
IV	13,582	1.6	6.9	11.3	5.5	38.2	1.5	2.4	38	58	21
V	23,464	1.6	7.6	12.0	7.2	54.3	1.7	2.6	12	65	19
VI	23,535	1.5	7.4	11.5	10.2	75.9	2.0	2.7	7	65	6
VII	23,957	1.4	7.7	10.8	6.5	50.0	1.9	2.7	13	64	0
VIII	17,014	1.4	7.5	10.3	6.5	49.1	1.4	2.2	16	47	18
IX	14,703	1.5	7.2	10.9	7.1	51.1	1.3	2.0	32	45	25

Creation of an organizational profile by facility and division including the multiple factors likely to influence productivity. Displayed separately are billable hour efficiency/organizational factors, staffing efficiency, and OR efficiency data.

services). Logically, to allow meaningful comparison of productivity, the work hours associated with these activities should be extracted when comparing tASA/FTE. Special consideration should be given to teaching activities especially in the context of Centers for Medicare & Medicaid Services/Medicare reimbursement. Studies have clearly demonstrated that the use of trainees is associated with financial benefits that need to be taken into consideration when considering overall efficiency.[12]

Productivity-Based Compensation

As early as 1936, incentive systems to improve worker productivity have been described in the medical literature[13] and a high percentage of anesthesiology departments currently use clinical incentive or productivity-based compensation plans.[1] These plans have been shown to be effective in increasing clinical work output including in previously published data from our department.[14,15] Productivity-based compensation plans are intended to differentiate workers by effort and efficiency; however, a multitude of factors beyond individual anesthesiologist control impact opportunities for tASA unit production. An understanding and an accounting of the impact of these factors can allow for adjustments to be made when comparing provider performance to allow for fair distribution within productivity-based compensation plans. Several examples from our own productivity-based compensation plan can demonstrate these necessary considerations. Within our plan, performance is based on comparison with a site-specific mean.[15] This recognizes organizational, staffing, and site-specific efficiency factors that impact productivity. Within complex sites comprised of subspecialty teams, we use an adjustment factor before calculation of incentive plan distribution to account for differences in opportunities available between teams. For example, Division I mean productivity by team is 19,622 for the general/trauma anesthesia team, 26,630 for the neuroanesthesiology team, 15,566 for the transplant team, and 16,462 for the cardiac team (see **Fig. 5**). Comparative mean performance of the general/trauma team to the others is used to calculate adjustment factors: general/trauma = 1, neuroanesthesiology = 0.74, transplant = 1.26, and cardiac = 1.19. The productivity of each individual anesthesiologist is then adjusted by this factor before final comparison and distribution within the performance-based compensation plan. We found these and other adjustments, when differential opportunity for productivity was apparent, to be a necessary administrative step to ensure fair distribution of compensation. A prerequisite to such adjustments is a knowledge and understanding of factors that contribute to differences in opportunity.

SUMMARY

Meaningful comparisons between anesthesiology groups or individuals is difficult because of the broad and varied differences in practice types and opportunity for tASA generation. Although attempts have been made using per case or per OR metrics by facility type, no two facilities are alike in the many factors that impact productivity opportunity. However, developing an organizational profile by facility or division that includes the multiple factors likely to influence productivity can provide considerable insight (**Table 5**). Additionally, a dynamic approach, with frequent tracking either monthly or quarterly, can allow for identification of trends and therefore tactical or operational changes to be made to improve productivity opportunity and encourage fairness throughout a system.

Because health care organizations use available anesthesiology productivity benchmarking data to compare providers and practices, a thorough understanding of factors impacting productivity opportunities is essential. Key stakeholders evaluating anesthesiology practice performance are generally unfamiliar with the differences between work relative value units and tASA productivity metrics and the factors influencing tASA opportunity. In our experience, educating our health care partners has become essential in working to achieve optimum efficiency. Although significant complexity exists, and impacting factors often overlap in influence, a model can be developed to evaluate the relative impact of each. This level of analysis and understanding of influencing factors should take place at the organizational level because it represents the prerequisite for any rational adjustments and meaningful comparisons between anesthesiology providers, divisions, or sites. Furthermore, this information allows for identification of organizational and facility opportunities for improved efficiency in the use of the resources of all surgical services.

ACKNOWLEDGMENTS

The authors thank William Thomson, MHA, MBA (Assistant Administrator, Department of Anesthesiology, University of Pittsburgh Medical Center) for collection and maintenance of faculty member data. The authors also thank Jim Ibinson, MD, PhD and Tetsuro Sakai, MD, PhD for statistical assistance and Jacques Chelly, MD, MBA for his editorial assistance with this article.

REFERENCES

1. Abouleish AE, Apfelbaum JL, Prough DS, et al. The prevalence and characteristics of incentive plans for clinical productivity among academic anesthesiology programs. Anesth Analg 2005;100(2):493–501.
2. Revicki DA, Orkin FK, Luce BR, et al. Physican payment reform: anesthesiology as a case study. Anesthesiology 1990;73(4):760–9.
3. Abouleish AE, Prough DS, Whitten CW, et al. The effects of surgical case duration and type of surgery on hourly clinical productivity of anesthesiologists. Anesth Analg 2003;97(3):833–8.
4. Abouleish AE, Prough DS, Barker SJ, et al. Organizational factors affect comparisons of the clinical productivity of academic anesthesiology departments. Anesth Analg 2003;96(3):802–12.
5. Hudson ME. Benchmarking anesthesiologists' performance: understanding factors that impact productivity. ASA Monitor 2016;80(6):40–2.
6. Feiner JR, Miller RD, Hickey RF. Productivity versus availability as a measure of faculty clinical responsibility. Anesth Analg 2001;93:313–8.
7. Sinclair DR, Lubarsky DA, Vigoda MM, et al. A matrix model for valuing anesthesia service with the resource-based relative value system. J Multidiscip Healthc 2014;7:449–58.
8. Abouleish AE, Prough DS, Whitten CW, et al. Increasing the value of time reduces the lost economic opportunity of caring for surgeries of longer-than-average times. Anesth Analg 2004;98(6):1737–42.
9. Giedraitis AV, Emerick TD, Nelson DF, et al. CRNA billed to staffed hours as a measure of operating room efficiency across a large multi-hospital health care system. American Society of Anesthesiologist Practice Management 2015. Atlanta (GA), October 24, 2015.p. A1280.
10. Nagretbetsky A, Gabriel RA, Dutton RP, et al. Growth of nonoperating room anesthesia care in the United States: a contemporary trends analysis. Anesth Analg 2017;124(4):1261–7.

11. Tsai MH, Huynh TT, Breidenstein MW, et al. A system-wide approach to physician efficiency and utilization rates for non-operating room anesthesia sites. J Med Syst 2017;41(7):112.
12. Backeris ME, Forte PJ, Beaman ST, et al. Financial implications of different interpretations of ACGME anesthesiology program requirements for rotations in the operating room. J Grad Med Educ 2013;5(2):315–9.
13. Incentives in industry. Br Med J 1936;1:318.
14. Reich DL, Galati M, Krol M, et al. A mission-based productivity compensation model for academic anesthesiology department. Anesth Analg 2008;107:1981–8.
15. Sakai T, Hudson M, Davis P, et al. Integration of academic and clinical performance based faculty compensation plans: a system and its impact on an anaesthesiology department. Br J Anaesth 2013;111(4):636–50.

Overlapping Surgery
A Case Study in Operating Room Throughput and Efficiency

Amanda J. Morris, MD[a],*, Joseph A. Sanford, MD[b],
Edward J. Damrose, MD[c], Samuel H. Wald, MD, MBA[a],
Bassam Kadry, MD[a], Alex Macario, MD, MBA[a]

KEYWORDS

- Concurrent • Efficiency • Metrics • Operations • Overlapping • Parallel • Surgery
- Throughput

KEY POINTS

- Fundamentals of OR management depend on optimal access, safety, efficiency, and throughput, and a keystone is proper allocation of OR time.
- Timely OR access is important to surgeons, so the opportunity cost of denying a surgeon's request to perform overlapping surgery must be considered.
- Published studies consistently lack higher adverse events for overlapping surgery, but overlap of "critical" portions of procedures should not occur and should be monitored.
- Overlapping surgery promotes efficiency when: surgeon idle time is costly, nonsurgical time is greater than surgical time, and surgeries can progress more in parallel.
- Overlapping surgery promotes throughput and productivity for: consistent, short-duration, and higher contribution margins per OR hour cases, and procedure lengthening is important.

The fundamentals of operating room (OR) management depend on developing policies and procedures that optimize access, safety, efficiency, throughput, and staff satisfaction. Later in this article, the authors present overlapping surgery as a case study toward these goals.

The authors have nothing to disclose.
[a] Department of Anesthesiology, Stanford Health Care, 300 Pasteur Drive H3580, Stanford, CA 94305, USA; [b] Department of Anesthesiology, University of Arkansas for Medical Sciences, 4301 West Markham, Little Rock, AR 72205, USA; [c] Division of Laryngology, Stanford Health Care, 801 Welch Road, Stanford, CA 94305, USA
* Corresponding author.
E-mail address: amandamd@stanford.edu

Anesthesiology Clin 36 (2018) 161–176
https://doi.org/10.1016/j.anclin.2018.01.002
anesthesiology.theclinics.com
1932-2275/18/© 2018 Elsevier Inc. All rights reserved.

MANAGEMENT GOALS FOR THE SURGICAL SUITE

The goals of OR management are inextricably linked. For example, increasing efficiency and throughput cannot come at the expense of patient safety. Increasing efficiency from the surgeon's perspective (maximal access and minimal nonsurgical time) must consider resultant inefficient use of other OR staff and their satisfaction. Increased efficiency may not translate to increased throughput and vice versa.

Given these multiple points of view, a starting point may be in the mathematical basis for the term OR inefficiency. OR inefficiency is defined by 2 crucial concepts: "overutilized and underutilized time" and ultimately is a function of the sum of these values[1] (**Table 1**). As the day of surgery approaches, the cost of underutilized OR time becomes negligible relative to the cost of overutilized time.[2]

Like the mathematical basis for OR inefficiency, there are agreed upon quantitative benchmarks for other measures that characterize optimally managed surgical faculties. From the example in **Table 1**, 10% to 20% excess staffing costs would reflect suboptimal OR management[3] (**Table 2**).

Because OR inefficiency is a function of overutilized and underutilized time, proper allocation of OR time is essential to efficiency. "Allocation" can be defined in the context of other important OR management terms (**Table 3**). Intuitively, this makes sense because if an OR is staffed for only 6 hours, yet the room consistently runs 9 hours, then this OR is not efficient. Because OR allocation is done months ahead of the day of surgery during tactical decision making, little can be done on the day of surgery to increase efficient use of OR staff.

Building upon the concepts of overutilized and underutilized time and allocated OR time, OR utilization reflects time that the OR is progressing with a case during allocated OR time. Herein, there are 2 ways of measuring utilization: "raw" versus "adjusted." "Raw utilization" equals proportion of allocated OR time that is taken up by hours of elective cases performed by a surgeon or surgical group during allocated OR time, excluding turnover times (**Fig. 1**). In other words, raw utilization reflects occupancy, not turnover times. On the other hand, "adjusted utilization" includes turnover time.[4]

Although efficiency focuses on minimizing overutilized and underutilized time and maximizing utilization during allocated OR time, throughput introduces an additional aim of maximizing number of cases. "Productivity" is the quotient of "throughput," that is, number of cases performed, over labor costs.[1] The distinction is important because an OR could be 100% efficient if zero cases were performed, so throughput, that is, performing cases, and more specifically productivity, which considers financial gains and losses of each case, must be higher priorities.

Table 1 Measures of operating room inefficiency	
Overutilized time	The hours that ORs run long. For example, if 12 h of cases (including turnovers) are performed with staff scheduled to work 10 h, there are 2 overutilized hours. The excess staffing cost is 40% (2 h/10 h = 20%, which is then multiplied by 2 to account for the overtime wages paid to late-staying staff and for the loss of staff due to poor morale and resulting recruitment costs for new staff)
Underutilized time	The hours a room finishes early and sits idle. If OR staff is scheduled to work from 7 AM to 5 PM, but the room finishes early at 4 PM, then there would be 1 h of underutilized time. The excess staffing cost would be 10% (1 h/10 h)

Table 2
A scoring system for OR efficiency

Metric	Points		
	0	1	2
Excess staffing costs	Greater than 10%	5–10%	Less than 5%
Start-time tardiness (mean tardiness of start times for elective cases per OR per day)	Greater than 60 min	45–60 min	Less than 45 min
Case cancellation rate	Greater than 10%	5–10%	Less than 5%
PACU admission delays (% of workdays with at least one delay in PACU admission)	Greater than 20%	10–20%	Less than 10%
Contribution margin (mean) per OR hour	Less than $1,000/h	$1,000–2,000/h	More than $2,000/h
Turnover times (mean setup and cleanup turnover times for all cases)	Greater than 40 min	25–40 min	Less than 25 min
Prediction bias (bias in case duration estimates per 8 h of OR time)	Greater than 15 min	5–15 min	Less than 5 min
Prolonged turnovers (% of turnovers that are more than 60 min)	Greater than 25%	10–25%	Less than 10%

Abbreviations: OR, operating room; PACU, postanesthesia care unit.
From Macario A. Are your hospital operating rooms "efficient"? A scoring system with eight performance indicators. Anesthesiology 2006;105(2):238; with permission.

OVERLAPPING SURGERY DEFINITIONS

The rationale behind allocating 2 ORs to a single surgeon for overlapping surgery is team based and based upon OR management goals, such as access, safety, efficiency, throughput, and productivity.

Table 3
Allocated operating room time and related operating room management definitions

Master surgical schedule	A cyclic timetable that defines number of ORs available, the open hours of the ORs, and the surgical groups given that OR time
Regularly scheduled hours	The hours that an OR team member plans on working on the days when not on call (eg, 7 AM to 5 PM)
Allocated OR time	Specific start and end times on a specific day of the week that is assigned to a surgical service (eg, the spine surgeons may be allocated OR time from 7 AM to 5 PM every Tuesday). This does not mean that additional cases would be turned away if the group could not finish them by 5 PM. Instead, OR time allocation indicates that the regularly scheduled hours planned for the surgeons are between 7 AM and 5 PM
Block time	A category of allocated OR time. Some surgical facilities decide that no case is scheduled into block time unless it can reasonably be expected to be finished within the block
Staffing	The process of calculating the number of OR teams that must be available at each time during the week. For example, there may be staffing for 4 ORs Monday through Thursday between 7 AM and 5 PM, and 7 AM to noon on Fridays

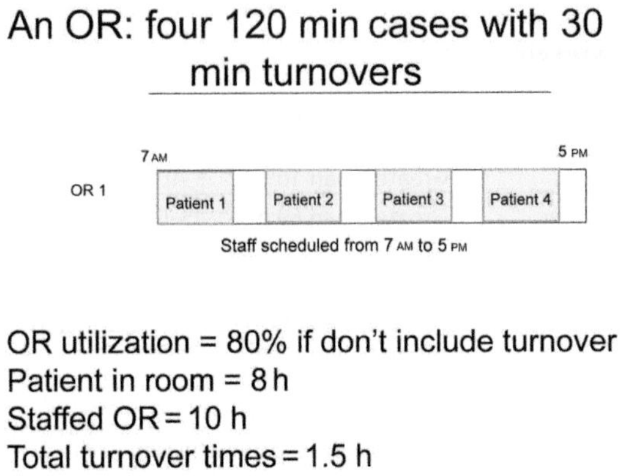

An OR: four 120 min cases with 30 min turnovers

OR utilization = 80% if don't include turnover
Patient in room = 8 h
Staffed OR = 10 h
Total turnover times = 1.5 h

Fig. 1. Raw versus adjusted utilization example whereby raw utilization equals 80% (8 hours of cases/10 hours staffed OR time) versus adjusted utilization equals 95% ([8 hours of cases + 1.5 hours of turnover time]/10 hours).

Conventionally, surgeons' cases are scheduled to run in series in 1 OR; however, this is not always the most effective use of resources because the OR is team based with processes that could be performed in parallel. For example, the patient needs to be transported into the OR, and anesthesia induction needs to be completed. The patient is then positioned on the OR bed, and only then can surgical incision commence. As such, there are periods of time when the surgeon is inactive. Overlapping surgery enables the surgeon to move directly from finishing critical portions in 1 procedure to starting critical portions in the next, minimizing surgeon downtime. For clarity, the American College of Surgeons (ACS) has provided precise definitions to be used in describing overlapping surgery[5] (**Table 4**).

As suggested, a challenge in discussing the complex topic of parallel surgery is the imprecision of terminology or the variety of scenarios that it entails. For example, a parallel surgery scenario could be "flipping rooms," in which overlap is confined to turnover time (ie, time between first patient out-of-room to next patient in-room within a single OR), such that there are never 2 patients in 2 ORs at the same time (**Fig. 2**A, Scenario 1). An alternative scenario could be overlap in turnover time plus

Table 4
Precise definitions regarding overlapping surgery as per the American College of Surgeons

Concurrent or simultaneous	Describes surgical procedures when the critical or key components of the procedures for which the primary attending surgeon is responsible are occurring all or in part at the same time
"Critical" or "key" portions	Describes stages of an operation when essential technical expertise and surgical judgment are necessary to achieve an optimal patient outcome. The critical or key portions are determined by the primary attending surgeon
"Overlapping or sequenced"	Describes the practice of the primary surgeon initiating and participating in another operation when he or she has completed the critical portions of the first procedure and is no longer an essential participant in the final phase of the first operation. These are by definition surgical procedures wherein key or critical portions of the procedure are occurring at different times

From American College of Surgeons. Statements on principles. 2016. Available at: https://www.facs.org/about-acs/statements/stonprin#definitions. Accessed November 7, 2017; with permission.

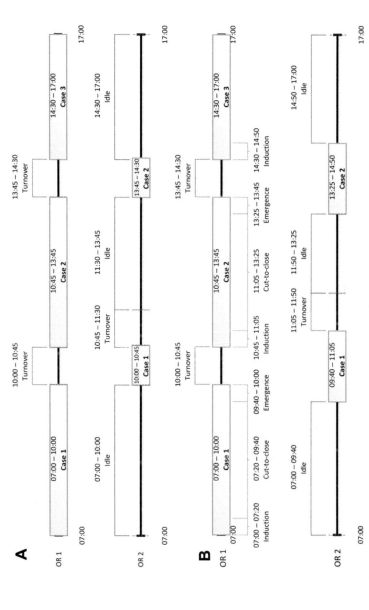

Fig. 2. Parallel room scenarios: (A) Scenario 1, (B) Scenario 2, (C) Scenario 3, and (D) Scenario 4.

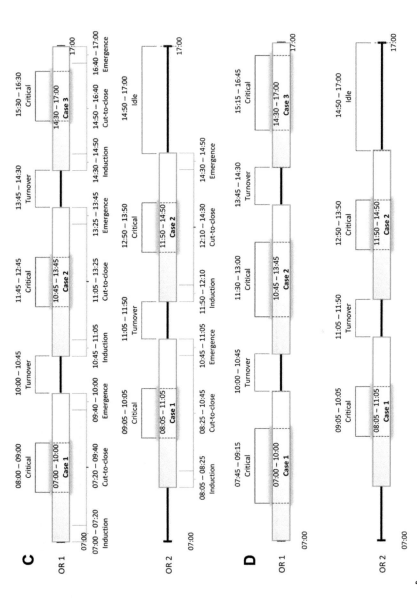

Fig. 2. (continued).

induction and emergence from anesthesia, such that the second patient is in the second room only during anesthesia-controlled time and turnover time in the first room and there never is an open wound in 2 patients in 2 ORs at the same time (**Fig. 2**B, Scenario 2). These scenarios are distinct from overlapping surgery and concurrent surgery (**Fig. 2**C, D, Scenarios 3 and 4, respectively). "Overlapping induction" is yet another term described in previous literature, which is distinct in that 1 room is assigned to a single surgeon, but anesthesia-controlled time occurs in parallel in a separate space from the OR. When a surgeon requests to run 2 rooms, hospitals need to assess the specific scenario involved.

Nationwide, the request by a surgeon to use 2 ORs in parallel for the purposes of efficiency and throughput is not uncommon. Although the precise frequency of overlapping surgery is unknown, when the Senate Finance Committee surveyed academic medical centers, 15 of 17 reviewed permitted it.[6] Similarly, a national survey of the American Academy of Otolaryngology found that 40% of surgeons reported some form of overlapping surgery.[7]

OVERLAPPING SURGERY AND OPERATING ROOM ACCESS

A major rationale for overlapping surgery is connected to the issue of OR access for surgeons, patients, and surgical trainees or qualified practitioners. Surgeons are reimbursed via a professional service fee on a per-case basis, and operating multiple rooms may allow a surgeon to complete more cases. The related issues of access and overlapping surgery may arise if a surgeon can regularly fill his or her block with cases and another OR is not fully utilized. Alternatively, a surgeon's request for a second room may conflict with another surgical service's block time, in which case a possible approach could be to compare quarterly or 6-month average utilization percentages, contribution margins (revenue minus variable costs), as well as strategic growth goals for each service. When a surgeon requests 2 rooms, the opportunity cost of denying a surgeon's request and losing the surgeon's business to a competing facility must be considered.

For surgeons in high demand, patient access to the ORs, that is, wait times for surgery, may be facilitated by this practice as well. It is generally assumed that patients would not support the concept of overlapping surgery and that the full attention of their surgeon is required throughout the case. In an ideal world, where there is unlimited access to surgeons and no wait time for surgery, perhaps this assumption holds true, but this is not certain. From a patient's perspective, for example, would a patient in pain, like from a broken hip, be willing to have parts of their surgery performed by trainee surgeons to have a hip replacement surgery done sooner and to stop the pain? Would a patient with unstable angina who needed coronary artery bypass grafting be willing to be the second patient in an overlapping room, knowing that the opening and closing of the procedure would start with trainees, but would be able to have the procedure weeks earlier, and potentially avoiding sudden death from acute coronary thrombosis? Would a patient with a rapidly growing malignancy be willing to get into the OR sooner, knowing the room overlaps with another case? Hospitals, communities, and society at large need to include these issues while discussing overlapping surgery.

Another consideration is the training of future generations of surgeons and the involvement of other qualified practitioners. The natural course of learning necessitates graduated degrees of responsibility. Overlapping surgery does not mean that the patient is abandoned to an unskilled practitioner. As an example, consider the closure of a wound and a trainee surgeon who requires twice as much time to close a wound as an attending surgeon, but the wound is effectively closed in both scenarios with no difference in outcome. Is this a price society would be willing to pay to add 1 more effective surgeon to its roster in the future? Furthermore, all members of the OR team ideally would practice at the top of their license, such that highly specialized members of the team would not be performing routine, technical tasks. Qualified practitioners, defined as 1 who is licensed to complete delegated portions of a procedure without direct supervision, can add value in this way.[5] The value of trainees and qualified practitioners contributing to the performance of overlapping surgery has implications for not only training and good organization but also costs.

OVERLAPPING SURGERY AND PATIENT SAFETY

Regardless of addressing OR access, no OR management strategy could persist if it compromised patient safety. That said, to date, 9 peer-reviewed studies comparing overlapping to nonoverlapping cases consistently demonstrate no significant differences across multiple patient safety measures.

A study at the Mayo Clinic drawing from University HealthSystem Consortium data (n = 26,725) and the ACS–National Surgical Quality Improvement Program (NSQIP) (n = 9349) found no difference in primary outcomes measures of 30-day mortality and length of stay (in 1 sample).[8] Similarly, another study evaluating NSQIP data involving 12,010 surgeries found no difference for death, serious morbidity, reoperation, or readmission.[9] Two tertiary-care institutions reviewing 1135 microvascular free flap surgeries found no difference in 30-day complications.[10] The same finding was present in a sample of 3640 sports medicine cases performed by 4 primary surgeons at an orthopedic surgical center.[11] Three studies from University of California in San Francisco examining vascular (N = 1219 by 1 surgeon), spine (N = 2319 by 3 surgeons), and neurosurgeries (N = 7358 by 9 surgeons) found no difference on most measures, including 30-day readmissions, length of stay, and estimated blood loss.[12–14] Another study on neurosurgery cases at the University of Utah (N = 1018 by 5 surgeons) lacked differences for any complications.[15] Most recently, another study focused on 14,872 neurosurgical cases at a single institution did not find differences for mortality or hospital readmission.[16]

Despite these consistent findings, study limitations must be considered. All the studies were nonrandomized involving a narrow group of procedure types or surgeons, and the definition of overlap may have included as little as 1 second accounting for some of the null findings, which illustrates the evolving definition of overlapping surgery and the need for continual monitoring.

Key to the safety of overlapping surgery is ensuring that overlap of critical portions of a procedure does not occur. "Concurrent surgery," in which the critical portions occur at the same time, is always inappropriate unless an emergency occurs elsewhere, whereas "overlapping surgery," in which critical portions do not occur at the same time, is permissible if the attending (or primary) surgeon:

1. Is present for all "critical" portions of the procedure;
2. Is immediately available to assist in the first room;
3. Designates a "qualified practitioner" to be physically present in the first room when not present.

These standards echo Center for Medicare and Medicaid (CMS) regulations for billing, such that a surgeon cannot bill and be reimbursed if the above requirements are not met.[17]

How best to define "critical" portions remains uncertain, however. Some have advocated leaving the decision to the attending surgeon, who understands the nuances and anticipated complications of the particular surgery, whereas others advocate oversight by an impartial multidisciplinary committee to minimize conflict of interest.[18] In reality, a solution that allows room for both may be most practical. Generally, CMS and the ACS state that opening and closing of the skin are considered noncritical.[5,17] Examples of critical portions could be the cutting or removal of a tumor in a cancer case, or the viewing of an organ in an endoscopic case, or placement of screws and fluoroscopy to confirm alignment in an orthopedic case. Essentially, "critical" implies the parts of the case that require the judgment or expertise of the primary attending surgeon.

To balance surgeon autonomy, patient safety, public accountability, and OR efficiency, there needs to be a reliable process for measuring "critical" periods of surgery, which might be left up to the attending surgeon (**Box 1**). Such a system for monitoring

---

Box 1
An outlined approach to monitor overlapping surgery

1. Is there a reliable process to measure "critical" periods of surgery, and can this process be reflected as a Key Performance Indicator that can be reported to leadership in terms of frequency of overlap and duration of overlap?
   a. If Yes, implement a policy to manage to these metrics.
   b. If No, then identify a process that can reliably capture the critical periods of surgery using reliable time stamp data.

2. Identify what time stamps are documented either electronically or on paper records:
   a. Patient room-in time
   b. Surgeon sign-in time
   c. Start of incision time
   d. Exposure complete time
   e. Start of closing time
   f. Surgeon sign-out time
   g. Operation-end time
   h. Patient room-out time

3. Identify which time stamps are reliably documented (**Table 5**).

4. For time stamps that are not entered regularly, consider proper training to enter the data (refer to step 7)

5. The choice of duration as will the definition of a "case," that is, patient room-in to patient room-out versus incision start to closure end, will impact both the frequency of overlap and duration of overlap (**Table 6**)

6. Develop a management policy and report to provide this data to leadership and surgeons

7. If training is not sufficient to fill in the data gap, consider an alternative time stamp
   a. To identify if time stamps are reliable, assess how complete the data are being used to measure period of overlap
   b. For systems on paper records, use anesthesia billing data as a source of information given that they will typically have time stamp data that may include anesthesia start, room-in, start of incision, room-out, and anesthesia end. These data are not optimal but can be used as a surrogate
   c. Keep in mind that with increased documentation burden, the likelihood of having complete and accurate data decreases. The process of choosing time stamps should take into consideration workflow logistics to improve the completeness and accuracy of data

Table 5
Sample results indicating frequency of time stamp documentation

	What Percent of Cases Have Both Time Stamps?
Patient room-in to patient room-out	99
Incision start to operation end	99
Incision start to start of closing	99
Exposure complete to start of closing	20
Surgeon sign-in to surgeon sign-out	50

could be used for reporting to hospital leadership as a Key Performance Indicator and for comparison with other quality metrics, such as patient safety indicators, to gauge the impact of overlapping surgery on surgical outcomes and postoperative complications. Monitoring would also be useful for professional billing because for both CMS and other private insurers, attending presence and participation in key portions are necessary for reimbursement.

PARALLEL ROOMS AND OPERATING ROOM EFFICIENCY

When access and safety have been established, assessing the impact of overlapping surgery on OR efficiency is key to sustainability of the practice. A motivation for overlapping surgery is decreasing overutilized time because in theory a surgeon's list of cases can be completed earlier in the day spread out in 2 rooms than they would be if done in series in 1 room. Meanwhile, it is possible underutilized time could increase if a set list of cases is spread out across 2 rooms rather than packed into 1 OR. Background literature specific to "overlapping surgery" and OR efficiency is limited and focuses more on "overlapping induction," but available evidence suggests that overlapping surgery promotes OR efficiency if a surgeon's idle time costs are high, the portion of parallelizability increases, surgical time is 2 hours or less, or the ratio of surgical to nonsurgical time is 1 or less.

Studies varying the ratio of surgeons to ORs (ie, "overlapping surgery") are limited, but 1 study by Batun and colleagues[19] uses mathematical modeling to determine the optimal number of ORs to open for 1 surgeon, considering different levels of turnover time (ranging from 0 to 2 times the original turnover time, which is 30 minutes) and parallelizable portions (ranging from zero to 1 times the original duration) for both high and low idle time costs ($88.74 and $17.75 per minute, respectively). As the parallelizable portion increases, so does the optimal number of ORs. For a given pair of turnover

Table 6
Examples of the choice of duration and the definition of a "case" impacting both the frequency of overlap and the duration of overlap

	Frequency of Overlap (%)	Duration of Overlap (% of Total Minutes of Case)
Patient room-in to patient room-out	15	7
Incision start to closure end	10	4
Incision start to closure start	7	3
Exposure complete to start of closing	2	1
Surgeon sign-in to surgeon sign-out	1	0.5

time and parallelizable proportions, the optimal number of ORs per surgeon is higher when surgeon idle costs are higher. In other words, the benefit of overlapping surgery becomes higher when surgeon idle costs are higher.

Studies varying ratio of OR anesthesia teams to ORs (ie, "overlapping induction") provide a related example on OR efficiency. A common finding in these studies was that overlapping induction reduced nonsurgical time and overtime but could increase idle time. Williams and colleagues[20] simulated 3 supervised anesthesia providers in 2 ORs (3:2) versus 2 supervised anesthesia providers in 2 ORs (2:2) and found that the 3:2 scenario significantly decreased certain nonsurgical periods, such as OR entry to surgical incision and post anesthesia care unit (PACU) transport to sign-out. However, 3:2 was not necessarily more efficient because even though overtime decreased, idle time increased (such that 2:2 was more cost-effective). Hanss and colleagues[21] also found that overlapping induction led to a decrease in nonsurgical time. Comparably, Brown and colleagues[22] found that overtime decreased (by 40 minutes per day per surgeon) during parallel processing of regional anesthesia.

Research into "overlapping induction" also has demonstrated that case duration influences OR efficiency. Marjamaa and colleagues[23] found that amount of underutilized time depended on whether short or long procedures were scheduled in parallel. Short procedures seemed to benefit most from staffed, individual induction rooms, that is, 4 ORs, 4 induction rooms, and 4 anesthesia teams. In contrast, central induction rooms, that is, 4 ORs, 1 central induction room, and 5 anesthesia teams worked best for long procedures. They also found that overutilized time was highest with a circulating induction team model, that is, 4 ORs, 4 induction rooms, and 5 anesthesia teams. This finding is consistent with other research suggesting that a surgical time of 2 hours or less or ratio of surgical to nonsurgical time of 1 or less supports the efficient use of parallel processing by minimizing downtime.[24,25] The basis of a shorter duration procedure or a case duration less than turnover time being helpful is that the greatest benefit of overlapping surgery occurs when there are a higher number of turnovers, thus a higher number of opportunities to minimize nonsurgical time with parallel processing.

It is worth pointing out that case variance also affects efficiency of parallel rooms. In a study on overlapping induction by Mulier and colleagues,[26] use of the anesthesia preparation room shortened nonoperative time. However, if there were switches in surgeons, anesthesiologists, or longer scheduled durations of the previous surgery, then nonoperative time increased. These findings suggest that efficiency can be determined by several factors related to case length variance.

PARALLEL ROOMS AND OPERATING ROOM THROUGHPUT AND PRODUCTIVITY

Minimizing underutilized and overutilized time with overlapping surgery is helpful for OR throughput if an additional case can be added during scheduled OR hours. Anecdotally, 1 surgeon in 1 room appears to have higher throughput than 1 surgeon in 2 rooms because the former is already 100% parallel and it is difficult to make up for downtime at the beginning and end of the parallel rooms. Again, available evidence focuses on both "overlapping surgery" and "overlapping induction," but in general, it appears that both can promote OR throughput and productivity depending on the specific case mix, case length, contribution margin.

Available literature specific to "overlapping surgery" and OR throughput suggests that there can be an increase in number of cases performed per day, particularly for high-volume, consistent, short-duration cases. Duffy[27] published a single surgeon's experience in increasing procedure volume of total joint arthroplasties (average tourniquet time: 35 minutes) from 250 to 750 per year over a 4-year time frame by dedicating 2 ORs for a single surgeon. The investigator emphasized the importance of a consistent surgical technique with little variance to improve speed of the procedure and of scheduling of complex cases with increased variance at the end of the day. Similarly, Natchiar and colleagues[28] studied high-volume cataract surgery and found that the number of operations per hour increased from 1 to 2 versus 6 to 8 for surgeons with 1 versus 2 operating tables, respectively. Marjamaa and colleagues[23] found that 3 surgeons divided among 4 ORs did not increase the number of cases performed in a day (but was more cost-effective).

Research on "overlapping induction" expands the topic further, combining throughput with cost analysis to determine that productivity generally improved but depended on the specifics of the OR model. For example, Marjamaa and colleagues[23] found greater productivity when there were individual induction rooms, a circulating induction team, and a central induction room. Stahl and colleagues[25] found that 1 central OR and attached induction and early recovery rooms resulted in greater throughput of 2 additional patients per day, mainly attributable to a reduction in nonsurgical time, and the typical net margins were greater than incremental costs. Furthermore, these profits would have been even greater if 1:1 anesthesia coverage were reduced to 1:2 according to a review of this study by Krupka and Sandberg.[29] Conversely, Hanss and colleagues[21] studied a 4-anesthesia-team-and-3-OR model and found that 2 more cases could be completed in a day with higher likelihood of profit than a traditional or 3-team-in-2-OR model, but the financial impact may have been overestimated according to Krupka and Sandberg.[29] Similarly, Williams and colleagues[20] found that 3-anesthesia-team-in-2-OR model was not more cost-effective than a 2:2 model.

OVERLAPPING SURGERY AND FINANCES

Thus, assessing 1-surgeon-in-2-OR model is primarily a financial calculation. There is no straightforward, 1-size-fits-all cost analysis that works for every hospital. Solutions need local assessment and customized intervention. For surgeons for whom the hospital is considering giving 2 ORs, the overall contribution margin per OR hour (total payment for hospital minus variable costs) for the elective cases should be calculated.[30] Following the Franklin Dexter financial lectures, consider the alterative OR as a pooled average among all surgeons who can operate in that space and then compare this to the contribution margin per OR hour for the surgeon requesting 2 rooms.[31,32]

Given that the approach above requires programming, statistics, and marketing analysis, to begin a preliminary financial calculation can serve to illustrate overlapping surgery's differential impact on contribution margin. Three scenarios are used:

1. 2 surgeons in 2 ORs (conventional, high-surgeon competition for ORs scenario);
2. 1 surgeon in 1 OR (conventional, low surgeon competition for ORs scenario);
3. 1 surgeon in 2 ORs (overlapping surgery case).

To simplify, assume identical case lengths and turnover times, an average hospital payer mix that results in a revenue of $5000 per case, surgeon reimbursement of $1500 per case, and an expense of $10,000 per open OR (assuming $1000 per OR hour for staffing and 10 hours of allocated OR time).

In the first scenario, multiple surgeons are completing for space, so 2 ORs are opened and there is 1 surgeon per OR. If each surgeon completes 3 cases (for a total of 6 cases in both ORs), then the hospital's profit is $10,000 ([Revenue of $5000 × 6 cases] − [Cost of $10,000 × 2 ORs]), and each surgeon would be reimbursed $4500 ($1500 × 3 cases).

In the second scenario, there is only 1 surgeon, and only 1 OR is opened. The surgeon in this scenario is different than the previous scenario in that he or she has more cases to complete or at least more OR time to complete them because there is low competition for OR time (assume 5 instead of 3 cases). The surgeon profits more ($7500), but the cost to the surgeon that he or she must stay later. The hospital also makes more ($15,000) and does not have the expense of opening another OR. This example ignores overtime costs.

Meanwhile, in the third overlapping surgery scenario, if the same surgeon in scenario 2 were offered a second OR and completed the 5 cases between 2 rooms, then the surgeon's profit would not change ($7500), and he or she would gain another benefit by not having to stay late. On the other hand, the hospital would profit the least amount compared with both previous scenarios ($5000) because of the cost associated with opening the second OR, but there are not as many cases performed as in the first scenario with 2 surgeons in 2 ORs.

These theoretic scenarios serve to illustrate typical financial driving forces for different stakeholders. As stated previously for a surgeon, an attraction of overlapping surgery is completing more cases in a shorter time. Hospitals will be weighing, "Is there empty space to grant a second OR to a single surgeon?," in which case hospitals may lose money ($5000 for the overlapping scenario vs $15,000 for the 1-surgeon-in-1-OR scenario) but not the surgeon's business. On the other hand, hospitals also will be weighing, "Would it be better to give the second OR to a second surgeon than to a single surgeon?," which can be more profitable ($10,000 for the 2-surgeons-in-2-ORs scenario vs $5000 for the overlapping scenario).

OVERLAPPING SURGERY AND OTHER CONSIDERATIONS INCLUDING PROCEDURE TIME

The limitation of the simplified explanation above is the financial result is dependent on multiple variables. As described in the OR efficiency and throughput sections of the article, the specifics on the ratios of surgeons to ORs, OR teams to ORs, ratio of case length to turnover time, and case length variance will ultimately influence the result. In addition, as suggested in the preliminary example above, contribution margin is key, which relies on relative value unit of the case, insurance reimbursement mix, and incremental cost of overhead for physical space.

How teams are compensated related to amount of downtime and overtime premiums also plays a role in costs. Although it may be difficult to quantify the cost for surgeon's downtime, productivity-based anesthesia groups will not be paid while sitting idle because of delay in a surgeon finishing the critical portions in another OR. Similarly, for an anesthesiologist salaried or employed by the hospital or for an anesthesia group with an exclusive contract with a hospital, it will likely be at the hospital's expense if the anesthesia teams are sitting idle. The same applies to nursing and other members of the OR team. Thus, hourly cost of underutilized and overutilized time is part of the equation for OR inefficiency, so compensation model of staff is an important factor.[33]

The amount of time it takes a procedure to be completed is another variable to be considered in the cost analysis.[34] There has been some evidence that procedure time is longer for overlapping cases. A study at the Mayo Clinic found that operative time for nonoverlapping cases was 85% of overlapping cases, which amounted to a median time of 40 minutes longer.[8] Similarly, investigators of a study on microvascular free flap cases found that procedure time of overlapping surgery was a mean of 21 minutes longer than nonoverlapping cases.[10]

Currently, the cause of longer procedure times in the setting of overlapping surgery is not fully understood, but several possibilities could be at play, including differences in definition of procedure time (eg, skin-to-skin vs patient room-in to room-out), involvement of other qualified practitioners, multidisciplinary overlapping operations involving multiple primary attending surgeons, and/or a phenomenon of case slowdown, namely less pressure to complete cases faster if the day will end earlier in 2 rooms with overlapping cases rather than 1 room with cases in series.

SUMMARY

OR efficiency and throughput are important in the OR suite because of the scarce resources that require coordination for the ORs to run efficiently. A key principle of OR management is to allocate the correct amount of OR time to each surgeon on each day of the week. The OR manager needs to work to understand their facility's data on utilization and other metrics because data become dialogue for change, such as responding to a request from a surgeon to run 2 rooms to improve surgeon, patient, and trainee access. Importantly, patient safety depends on critical parts not overlapping, which can be monitored through a novel, stepwise approach introduced in this article. Overlapping surgery promotes OR efficiency and throughput if a surgeon's idle time costs are high, the portion of parallelizability increases, surgical time is 2 hours or less, or the ratio of surgical to nonsurgical time is 1 or less and particularly for high-volume surgeons with consistent, short-duration cases and higher contribution margins per OR hour than a pooled average of other surgeons combined. The influence of procedure times will be an important factor in determining the impact of overlapping surgery on OR throughput and efficiency.

REFERENCES

1. McIntosh C, Dexter F, Epstein RH. The impact of service-specific staffing, case scheduling, turnovers, and first-case starts on anesthesia group and operating room productivity: a tutorial using data from an Australian hospital. Anesth Analg 2006;103(6):1499–516.

2. Macario A. Implementing operating room management science: from the bench to the scheduling office. Eur J Anaesthesiol 2014;31(7):355–60.

3. Macario A. Are your hospital operating rooms "efficient"? A scoring system with eight performance indicators. Anesthesiology 2006;105(2):237–40.

4. Macario A. The limitations of using operating room utilisation to allocate surgeons more or less surgical block time in the USA. Anaesthesia 2010;65(6):548–52.

5. Statements on principles. American College of Surgeons; 2016. Available at: https://www.facs.org/about-acs/statements/stonprin#definitions. Accessed November 7, 2017.

6. Senate Finance Committee Concurrent and Overlapping Surgeries Report Final.pdf. Senate Finance Committee Report. 2016. Available at: https://www.finance.senate.gov/imo/media/doc/Concurrent%20Surgeries%20Report%20Final.pdf. Accessed November 7, 2017.

7. Cognetti DM, Nussenbaum B, Brenner MJ, et al. Current state of overlapping, concurrent, and multiple-room surgery in otolaryngology: a national Survey. Otolaryngol Head Neck Surg 2017. https://doi.org/10.1177/0194599817723897.

8. Hyder JA, Hanson KT, Storlie CB, et al. Safety of overlapping surgery at a high-volume referral center. Ann Surg 2017;265(4):639–44.

9. Liu JB, Berian JR, Ban KA, et al. Outcomes of concurrent operations: results from the American College of Surgeons' National Surgical Quality Improvement Program. Ann Surg 2017. https://doi.org/10.1097/SLA.0000000000002358.
10. Sweeney L, Rosenthal EL, Light T, et al. Effect of overlapping operations on outcomes in microvascular reconstructions of the head and neck. Otolaryngol Head Neck Surg 2017;156(4):627–35.
11. Zhang AL, Sing DC, Dang DY, et al. Overlapping surgery in the ambulatory orthopaedic setting. J Bone Joint Surg 2016;98(22):1859–67.
12. Zygourakis CC, Lee J, Barba J, et al. Performing concurrent operations in academic vascular neurosurgery does not affect patient outcomes. J Neurosurg 2017. https://doi.org/10.3171/2016.6.JNS16822.
13. Zygourakis CC, Sizdahkhani S, Keefe M, et al. Comparison of patient outcomes and cost of overlapping versus nonoverlapping spine surgery. World Neurosurg 2017. https://doi.org/10.1016/j.wneu.2017.01.064.
14. Zygourakis CC, Keefe M, Lee J, et al. Comparison of patient outcomes in 3725 overlapping vs 3633 nonoverlapping neurosurgical procedures using a single institution's clinical and administrative database. Neurosurgery 2017;80(2):257–68.
15. Guan J, Brock AA, Karsy M, et al. Managing overlapping surgery: an analysis of 1018 neurosurgical and spine cases. J Neurosurg 2016. https://doi.org/10.3171/2016.8.JNS161226.
16. Bohl MA, Mooney MA, Sheehy JP, et al. Overlapping surgeries are not associated with worse patient outcomes: retrospective multivariate analysis of 14 872 neurosurgical cases performed at a single institution. Neurosurgery 2017. https://doi.org/10.1093/neuros/nyx472.
17. Medicare claims processing manual - Clm104c12.Pdf. Available at: https://www.cms.gov/Regulations-and-Guidance/Guidance/Manuals/downloads/clm104c12.pdf. Accessed November 7, 2017.
18. Mello MM, Livingston EH. The evolving story of overlapping surgery. JAMA 2017. https://doi.org/10.1001/jama.2017.8061.
19. Batun S, Denton BT, Huschka TR, et al. Operating room pooling and parallel surgery processing under uncertainty. INFORMS J Comput 2011;23(2):220–37.
20. Williams BA, Starling SL, Bircher NG, et al. Optimization of anesthesia staffing using simulation modeling. Am J Anesthesiol 1998;25:113–20.
21. Hanss R, Buttgereit B, Tonner PH, et al. Overlapping induction of anesthesia: an analysis of benefits and costs. Anesthesiology 2005;103(2):391–400.
22. Brown MJ, Subramanian A, Curry TB, et al. Improving operating room productivity via parallel anesthesia processing. Int J Health Care Qual Assur 2014;27(8):697–706.
23. Marjamaa RA, Torkki PM, Hirvensalo EJ, et al. What is the best workflow for an operating room? A simulation study of five scenarios. Health Care Manag Sci 2009;12(2):142–6.
24. Harders M, Malangoni MA, Weight S, et al. Improving operating room efficiency through process redesign. Surgery 2006;140(4):509–16.
25. Stahl JE, Sandberg WS, Daily B, et al. Reorganizing patient care and workflow in the operating room: a cost-effectiveness study. Surgery 2006;139(6):717–28.
26. Mulier JP, De Boeck L, Meulders M, et al. Factors determining the smooth flow and the non-operative time in a one-induction room to one-operating room setting. J Eval Clin Pract 2015;21:205–14.
27. Duffy GP. Maximizing surgeon and hospital total knee arthroplasty volume using customized patient instrumentation and swing operating rooms. Am J Orthop 2011;40(11 suppl):5–8.

28. Natchiar G, Thulasiraj RD, Sundaram RM. Cataract surgery at Aravind Eye Hospitals: 1988-2008. Community Eye Health 2008;21(67):40–2.
29. Krupka DC, Sandberg WS. Operating room design and its impact on operating room economics. Curr Opin Anaesthesiol 2006;19(2):185–91.
30. Macario A. Hospital profitability per hour of operating room time can vary among surgeons. Anesth Analg 2001;93:669–75.
31. Dexter F. Operating room financial assessment for tactical decision making (allocating 'block time'). University of Iowa Division of Management Consulting Education in Operating Room Management; 2017. Available at: http://www.franklindexter.net/Lectures/FinancialTalk.pdf. Accessed November 8, 2017.
32. Dexter F. Strategic planning: financial impact of different types of surgery. University of Iowa Division of Management Consulting Education in Operating Room Management; 2017. Available at: http://www.franklindexter.net/Lectures/StrategicFinancial.pdf. Accessed November 8, 2017.
33. Macario A. What does one minute of operating room time cost? J Clin Anesth 2010;22(4):233–6.
34. Macario A. Truth in scheduling: is it possible to accurately predict how long a surgical case will last? Anesth Analg 2009;108(3):681–5.

Section II: Quality and Reporting

Measuring Quality for Individual Anesthesia Clinicians

John Allyn, MD*, Craig Curry, MD

KEYWORDS

- Quality improvement • Quality management system (QMS)
- Quality data collection and reporting • Physician measurement
- Privileging: ongoing professional practice evaluation • Safety culture

KEY POINTS

- The quality management system (QMS) must have a system focus. Measuring quality for individual anesthesia clinicians should occur at the system level.
- Provider-specific outcome measures should be avoided.
- Quality data must not be used for provider privileging.
- A strong safety culture provides the foundation for a robust QMS.

INTRODUCTION

For more than 20 years, our private group has collected data about the anesthesia experience of our patients. In the early years, our focus was on data collection and how to do this effectively and efficiently. Over time, we began to analyze our data and address system issues to improve our care of patients. The discussion that follows discusses core principles that should guide the quality management system (QMS), how the work is done, and examples of challenges and successes along the way.

Our educational goals for this article are to help readers to understand the following:

- How to collect and report data to anesthesia clinicians
- Why quality data should be separate from privileging data
- Why outcome measures are not useful at the individual provider level
- Meaningful use for the QMS and how these data allow groups of anesthesia clinicians to demonstrate their value to the facilities at which they work

---

Disclosure Statement: Drs J. Allyn and C. Curry are employed by Spectrum Healthcare Partners, which markets a quality-improvement tool, FIDES.
Department of Anesthesiology and Peri-operative Medicine, Spectrum Healthcare Partners, Maine Medical Center, 22 Bramhall Street, Portland, ME 04102, USA
* Corresponding author.
E-mail address: allynj@spectrummg.com

Anesthesiology Clin 36 (2018) 177–189
https://doi.org/10.1016/j.anclin.2018.01.003   **anesthesiology.theclinics.com**

- How a strong safety culture and multidisciplinary quality improvement (QI) committee supports the QMS

DATA COLLECTION AND REPORTING

Our original data collection tools were paper based. These collection tools were developed for providers to use at the point of care and were designed to minimize disruption of work flow to maximize completion rates; this was reported by providers as critical to gaining acceptance and participation with data collection. Preformatted forms with unique case identification codes were attached to each anesthetic record, which contained the same identifier. Billing information, which contained many critical quality data elements, including providers' names, time and duration of case, and specific *Current Procedural Terminology* (*CPT*) codes, was abstracted from the clinical record and linked back to each case using the unique case identification code, thus, reducing any redundant data entry required at the point of care. Data elements actually collected on the form were limited elements of care not available in the billing extract, such as medications used during cases and clinical outcome indicators. Originally, the clinical outcome indicators were developed through an internal consensus process and gradually became based on literature and recommendations from the Anesthesia Quality Institute and the National Anesthesia Clinical Outcomes Registry.[1] At sites of service where we have converted from paper charts to an electronic health record (EHR), we changed to an integrated electronic data collection form that is launched from within the EHR; this was in keeping with our principle of minimizing the disruption of workflow. Case identification information is extracted from the EHR as the form is launched, which again allows us to gather quality data from our billing files and link them to the quality data gathered on the data form. Our ultimate goal is to extract all our quality data directly from the EHR; presently, we are extracting time, medication, and some clinical outcomes, such as temperatures, blood sugars, and postoperative pain scores, as has been described elsewhere.[2] We continue to rely on our quality data entry tool for other clinical outcome indicators, such as possible aspiration, myocardial infarction, and new neurologic injury, which are not as easily extracted from the clinical record (refer to **Table 1**). Also, using a self-reported quality data collection tool separate from the clinical record likely provides for collection of data unique from that which can be directly extracted from the clinical record, including text comments that are not part of the medical record. Studies have shown more adverse outcomes may be identified using self-reported quality tools than are extracted from the medical record by chart reviews.[3,4] The reasons for this are multifactorial but likely include fear of litigation from reporting such events in the medical record. Although underreporting is always a concern, we have used methods to increase our reporting, including a strong culture of safety that emphasizes frequent feedback and system-based improvements over individual blame or accountability. These principles have recently been shown to substantially improve incident reporting at one institution.[5]

We also provide continuous feedback at the individual provider, service line, and site of service levels. Feedback at every level is critical to the success of any program. Individual provider reports are provided annually and on request. This information serves to motivate individuals to participate fully in the collection of the data and allows them to reflect on their own practice. Providing individual feedback of this nature has been shown to encourage behaviors that can lead to improved participation and outcomes.[6,7] Aggregate service line and site of service level reports allow respective clinical directors, committees, and administrators to assess the ongoing

Table 1
Sources of data included in the quality management system

From EHR Extract	From Billing	From Data Form
Induction agent	Facility identification	Actual disposition from OR
Intraoperative anesthetic or sedative	Date of service	Airway management
Muscle relaxant	Patient name	Intraoperative observations
Reversal given	Date of birth	Postanesthesia observations
Intraoperative beta-blocker	Sex	Discharge delay
Intraoperative analgesic	Surgical *CPT* code	Intraoperative warming
Preoperative or intraoperative antiemetic	Anesthesia *CPT* code	Free text comments
Start anesthesia time	Concurrency	
End anesthesia time	Billing modifiers	
Start surgical time	*ICD-9/ICD-10* No. 1: primary diagnosis	
End surgical time	Physical status classification (ASA)	
Blood sugar (preoperative, intraoperative, PACU)	Primary anesthesia type	
Postanesthesia core temp	Surgeon name	
NRS (preoperative, PACU)	Primary anesthesia provider Name	
Postanesthesia vomiting	Second anesthesia provider Name (ie resident, CRNA, AA, SRNA)	
Postanesthesia antiemetic		

Abbreviations: AA, anesthesia assistant; ASA, American Society of Anesthesiologists; CRNA, certified registered nurse anesthetist; ICD-9, International Classification of Diseases, Ninth Revision; ICD-10, International Classification of Diseases, Tenth Revision; NRS, numeric rating scale; OR, operating room; PACU, postanesthesia care unit; SRNA, student registered nurse anesthetist; temp, temperature.

performance in their respective areas while also demonstrating the value of the QMS to the institution as a whole. These reports are reviewed more frequently, as the aggregate numbers allow for more meaningful assessments at shorter intervals. For example, **Fig. 1** tracks our postoperative vomiting rate for all patients over the last 17 years and **Fig. 2** shows individual provider feedback compared with the peer group.

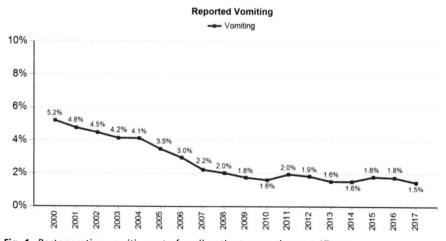

Fig. 1. Postoperative vomiting rate for all patients over the past 17 years.

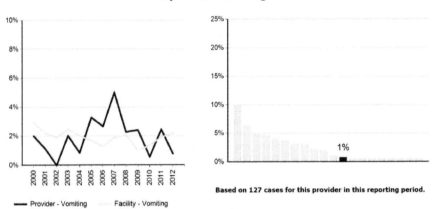

Fig. 2. Individual provider feedback (vomiting rate) compared with the group's average over several years. The vomiting rate for the current year is shown for all providers with the individual provider identified by the dark blue bar.

Our completion rates for quality data forms vary by phase of care and site of service. The intraoperative portion of the form is completed by the providers caring for patients in the operating room (OR). We began by providing private feedback of each individual's rate of completion compared with his or her peers. As the providers became comfortable with the process, we began providing open feedback on rates of return. Finally, as a group, we chose to set a minimum rate of completion as one of our Ongoing Professional Practice Evaluation (OPPE) criteria: failure to meet this minimum would result in a focused provider performance evaluation. Since we began using this as an OPPE criterion, all of our providers have been able to meet the requirement. With each step there was a progressive increase in completion rates, and presently our OR phase rates of completion are all more than 90% for all providers and at each site of service. The postanesthesia care unit (PACU) phase is typically completed by nurses caring for patients in the recovery room. These rates vary more considerably by site of service, ranging from 40% to more than 90%. This variation is likely related to perceived value to the nurses at each site as well as lack of clear attribution for responsibility and direct feedback about completion rates. We have worked to improve our returns by providing reports on our use of the data provided to us on improving care that has been effective at some sites.

We also use these data for critical incident and quantitative reviews. For critical incident reviews, we have identified indicators that trigger in-depth case reviews that are presented at a monthly committee meeting. These meetings are multidisciplinary and include surgical and anesthesia staff. The focus of these reviews is to identify system-based opportunities to prevent similar events from occurring. These reviews have led to many changes in our department, including implementation of crisis checklists, massive transfusion protocols, and improved communication tools for anesthesia providers. For quantitative reviews, we mine our quality data for variance in outcomes and then look for relevant associations that may allow us to explain this variability as well as suggest system changes to improve our outcomes. In one such example, we identified an association between an increased rate of reintubation and our use of rocuronium; we educated our providers about this association and reduced our rates of reintubation. We have also used quantitative reviews to demonstrate success with changes in our practice. For example, we were able to show a dramatic reduction in pain requiring intervention in our PACUs by implementing a preoperative block program for our joint service. Because of our ability to demonstrate its effectiveness in our own practice, that block program was adopted hospital wide.

WHY QUALITY DATA SHOULD BE SEPARATED FROM PRIVILEGING DATA

Although the questions make sense, which anesthesiologist has the lowest morbidity (eg, nausea) or mortality rate, we lack an answer for several reasons. These reasons include insufficient individual case and outcome numbers and lack of valid risk-adjustment tools. Even expensive and statistically rigorous studies of high-rate providers in high-risk cases, such as cardiac anesthesia, have been unable to identify outliers based on such objective outcomes as mortality.[8,9] Although data collected for QI is sufficient for developing a hypothesis about an individual provider or a group's practice, studies such as these cast a sobering light on using such data with less sophisticated assessments to compare providers in any accountable fashion.

Chance (anticipated random variation) must also be considered, especially when considering low-frequency events (eg, mortality).[10] Even when looking at system or hospital performance, there are challenges. For example, a hospital's National Surgical Improvement Project ranking for a procedure may not predict future performance.[11] This concern is especially an issue for low-volume procedures (eg, esophagectomies for many hospitals), as by chance alone a hospital's performance is more likely to be low or high reflecting a larger standard error of the mean (ie, the expected variability for a low-volume center will be higher).[12] Finally, attempts at assigning outcomes to individual providers are too costly. Resources are limited, and failure to use the allocated resources well may harm the QMS.[13] The QMS must maintain a system focus.

Although the discussion describes a reason why the QMS should not waste resources on assigning outcome measures to individual providers, the primary reason for maintaining a system focus is that this is where most of the opportunities for improvement reside.[14] Stated differently, using outcome measures to weed out bad apples is not possible; even if it were, the expense associated with this work would miss the largest opportunities for improvement, addressing system issues. There is one exception to this statement: individuals who are disrespectful and disruptive to your organization's safety culture must be removed. These individuals will be identifiable through reporting systems outside your QMS (more on this topic in the privileging and safety culture sections).

The Centers for Medicare and Medicaid Services (CMS), and those with deemed-status to accredit hospitals or facilities for the CMS, require provider-specific measures as a means to justify initial, new, or ongoing privileges for providers. For example, the Joint Commission uses Focused Professional Practice Evaluation (FPPE) and OPPE.[15]

Avoid the use of QMS measures to support provider privileging. Our concern is that, lacking data for individual providers, systems will look to the QMS for these data. We think this behavior puts the QMS at risk. In addition, to identify system problems, the QMS needs individuals to feel safe in reporting concerns. If some of these issues are then used as privileging measures (ie, are potentially punitive), individuals will cease to report them; this worry has been described earlier by others.[13] The airline industry supports 2 separate systems to accomplish the goals of identifying concerns to improve the system (ie, QMS work) and to meet regulatory requirements for public reporting (ie, provider privileging).[16]

Maintain separate systems for anesthesia providers and system concerns. As depicted in the attached diagram (**Fig. 3**), our privileging measures are not provided by our QMS. The one exception, and the only data moving outside the QMS to the provider privileging area, is a provider's participation rate in the QMS. Years ago, we set the expectation that all our providers must participate (fill out the forms on paper or electronically for all of their cases) in our QMS. Therefore, as discussed previously, when choosing provider-specific measures, we decided to monitor the individual provider participation rate in our QMS (**Fig. 4**). We do allow data to flow from the provider-privileging system to our QMS; for example, a sentinel event involving a provider would also inform the QMS to make sure that system issues were identified and responded to appropriately. A copy of the OPPE metrics we use today is attached (**Fig. 5**) along with an example of our FPPE (**Fig. 6**) for new providers. These metrics apply for all individuals with core (general) privileges; providers seeking or maintaining noncore privileges (specialty, eg, pediatric or pain) will also require FPPE and OPPE metrics to justify the noncore privileges. The Joint Commission provides examples for OPPE measures ("Medical Staff" chapter 08.01.03).[15] Some of their suggestions are outcome measures, which should be avoided as discussed previously, and others lack a means of robust risk adjustment (eg, use of consultants, length-of-stay data). In addition, the use of these outcome measures may negatively impact care, as providers or systems may avoid providing care to the sickest patients.[17]

SAFETY CULTURE

Whether an organization is able to collect data, support open discussion about system performance, and implement QI initiatives will depend heavily on the organization's leadership and the strength of its safety culture. All caregivers must feel they have a voice and must feel safe when reporting concerns. A strong safety culture is blame free in its analysis of system performance and methods to reduce human error. To establish and maintain the trust of all caregivers, individuals must be held accountable for their behaviors by a process that is equitable for all caregivers.

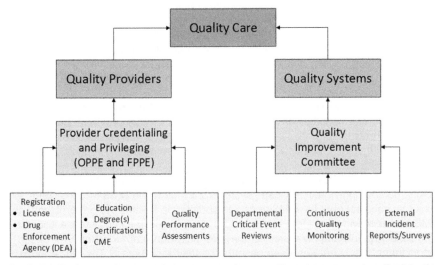

Fig. 3. Privileging measures are kept separate from quality measures as described in the text. Both the provider privileging process and the quality management system work to continuously improve the care of our patients. CME, continuing medical education.

Provider Completion Rate

All Facilities
All Service Lines
All Providers

Reporting Period: January 2017 - August 2017

Physician Completion Rate - All Cases

Provider	ADF Received	ADF Sections Completed	ADF Sections Available	Percent Completed (0%–100%)
	301	4,077	4,104	99%
	456	1,376	1,390	99%
	344	4,543	4,607	99%
	279	2,820	2,867	98%
	499	9,009	9,166	98%
	251	3,377	3,437	98%
	251	3,212	3,272	98%
	292	3,592	3,670	98%
	286	3,785	3,872	98%
	552	8,077	8,268	98%
	100	1,464	1,500	98%
	829	10,704	10,988	97%
	348	5,056	5,198	97%
	884	11,153	11,482	97%
	303	3,929	4,055	97%
	141	2,285	2,359	97%
	948	12,110	12,576	96%
	917	11,305	11,760	96%
	321	3,617	3,765	96%
	591	6,412	6,687	96%
	219	2,949	3,090	95%
	1,036	12,645	13,258	95%
	206	3,040	3,190	95%
	563	8,480	8,902	95%
	665	9,718	10,224	95%
	523	7,888	8,305	95%
	792	10,038	10,576	95%
	217	3,461	3,648	95%
	305	4,294	4,529	95%
	305	4,472	4,717	95%
	978	11,845	12,511	95%
	302	4,427	4,677	95%
	360	5,546	5,863	95%
	254	3,718	3,932	95%
	758	10,211	10,803	95%

This record is maintained as part of either (1) a hospital quality program for the identification and prevention of medical injury (including education) pursuant to the Maine Health Security Act (24 MRSA, Chapter 21) or (2) a confidential quality improvement program involving review of medical care on the behalf of physicians, conducted under the auspices of the Maine Medical Association as authorized under the provisions of 31 MRSA, Section 3296

Fig. 4. The report shows individual provider participation rates (the percentage of data fields that were completed) in our QMS. Overall the participation rate is very high.

An organization's culture has been described as the byproduct of the actions of the organization that are demonstrated consistently on a daily basis.[18] These behaviors depend greatly on the behaviors of the organization's leadership. Words whisper, actions thunder: if leadership states patient safety is its first priority and behaves daily as if OR efficiency is its focus, the culture of the organization will reward efficiency ahead of patient safety priorities.

Ongoing Professional Performance Evaluation

, MD
Licensure Date:

Anesthesia South Subspecialty:	LEGEND		
	Adequate	Request for Improvement	Inadequate
Patient Care:	**MEASURE:**	**Outcome:**	Recommended Action(s):
	Malpractice Cases & Board of Licensure Complaints	No claims in the past 10 y or BOL complaints	
Practitioners are expected to provide patient care that is compassionate, appropriate, and effective for the promotion of health, prevention of illness, treatment of disease and care at the end of life.	**MEASURE:**	**Outcome:**	Recommended Action(s):
	Mandated Sentinel Events (JC & State of ME)	No reported sentinel events	
	MEASURE:	**Outcome:**	Recommended Action(s):
	Anesthetic Case Count Cardiac - 25 CPB per year Pediatric - 12 cases/year under age 1	# of Cases:	
Professionalism:	**MEASURE:**	**Outcome:**	Recommended Action(s):
Practitioners are expected to demonstrate behaviors that reflect a commitment to continuous professional development, ethical practice, and understanding and sensitivity to diversity and a responsible attitude toward their patients, their profession and society.	Event Tracking	No reported events exhibiting a pattern.	
Interpersonal & Communication Skills:	**MEASURE:**	**Outcome:**	Recommended Action(s):
Practitioners are expected to demonstrate interpersonal and communication skills that enable them to establish and maintain professional relationships with patients, families and other members of health care teams.	Physician 360 Feedback Program	360 Professional Development survey completed in date with # participants. The feedback will go to the provider in date. Date of next survey is date.	
Medical/Clinical Knowledge:	**MEASURE:**	**Outcome:**	Recommended Action(s):
	CME & Subspecialty Specific Credits Cardiac - Presents at 1 MMC Cardiac Conference Per Year Pain - National Pain Meeting every 3 y Pediatric - Obtain subspecialty specific CME and SIM training and attend a nationally recognized pediatric anesthesia, critical care, or congenital cardiac meeting every two years	Met the State of Maine requirement for last license renewal in 2016. Next renewal is in 2017.	
	MEASURE:	**Outcome:**	Recommended Action(s):
	Maintenance of Certification (MOC) Pain - MOC grace period of 12 mo Pediatric - Board Certification in Pediatric Anesthesia by 1/2016 or within 3 years of completion of Fellowship in Pediatric Anesthesia		
Practitioners are expected to demonstrate knowledge of established and evolving biomedical, clinical and social sciences and the application of their knowledge to patient care and the education of others.	**MEASURE:**	**Outcome:**	Recommended Action(s):
	Meeting Attendance & Compliance w/ Mandatory Trainings Annual Compliance Training: Bi-Weekly Cardiac Conferences:	Completed	
	MEASURE:	**Outcome:**	Recommended Action(s):
	Advanced Cardiac Life Support (ACLS) / Pediatric Advanced Life Support (PALS) Certification, Current	ACLS renews in	
	Testamur or certification in Advanced Perioperative TEE	PALS renews in	
	MEASURE:	**Outcome:**	Recommended Action(s):
	MMC - eLearn for CLABSI	Passed	
	MMC - Proctored Insertion	Passed	
Practice-Based Learning & Improvement:	**MEASURE:**	**Outcome:**	Recommended Action(s):
Practitioners are expected to be able to use scientific evidence and methods to investigate, evaluate and improve patient care.	Participation in Quality Programs Implemented by the Department	Completing Anesthesia Data Form in physician only cases: 2016 # cases completed = % 2017 # cases completed = %	
System-Based Practice:	**MEASURE:**	**Outcome:**	Recommended Action(s):
	Compliance with Anesthesia Care Standards	Not a statistical outlier for 2015 – 2017	
Practitioners are expected to demonstrate both an understanding of the contexts and systems in which health care is provided and the ability to apply this knowledge to improve and optimize healthcare.	**MEASURE:**	**Outcome:**	Recommended Action(s):
	Narcotic Reconciliation Documentation	No Reports	
	MEASURE:	**Outcome:**	Recommended Action(s):
	Regional & National Initiatives	Met 2016 reporting via the MaineHealth Accountable Care Organization as a participant in the Medicare Shared Savings Program	

Applicants statement that no health problems exist that could affect his or her practice.

Fig. 5. The ongoing professional performance evaluation metrics used currently by the Spectrum Medical Group are shown. The metrics are grouped by the competency being assessed (eg, professionalism).

CONFIDENTIAL PROFESSIONAL COMPETENCE/QUALITY REVIEW MATERIAL
DO NOT DUPLICATE OR DISTRIBUTE
CONFIDENTIAL

Date: [DATE]

To: Peer Review File

Re: [NAME]

Focused Professional Performance Evaluation (FPPE) is a process whereby an organization evaluates the professional privilege specific performance of a practitioner. Upon appointment, the FPPE is implemented for a time-limited period for all new clinical staff members and may also be applied in evaluation of active clinical staff members.

The intent is to review and improve care, identify educational needs of new staff members and help new staff members comply with complex documentation requirements and adhere to practice culture. Currently the FPPE includes a review of the following areas:

Patient Care

- Malpractice Cases in the past 10 y for evidence of unusual patterns or an excessive number resulting in final judgments against the applicant.
  - ***Result: No reported cases.***

Interpersonal and Communication Skills

- Physician 360 feedback survey participation in receiving the feedback from peers at 6 mo
  - ***Result: This review took place on [date], with [#] responses.***

Medical/Clinical Knowledge

- 10 cases for completeness, appropriateness of care, accuracy and clarity in the following areas: Pre-anesthetic care, immediate pre-induction assessment, details of the anesthetic management, adherence to clinical protocols, post anesthesia care
  - ***Result:***
- Confirmation of ACLS/PALS certification
  - ***Result:***
- Compliance with Central line privileging criteria of demonstrating 10 insertions, and 1 observed insertion, and Completion of the CLABSI Prevention Learning Module
  - ***Result:***
    - ***Case Count: #***
    - ***eLearn: Passed or Failed***
    - ***Proctored Insertion: Completed or Not Completed***
- Documentation of completion of mandatory compliance training, clinical orientation is at all anesthetizing locations and *CRNA Scope of Practice Orientation*
  - ***Result: Documentation is on file, completed all necessary Training and Orientation.***

Practice-Based Learning and Improvement

- Individual QI report for participation and completeness of the Anesthesia Data Form
  - ***Result: Participation % from date-date***
- New anesthesiologists are required to attend regularly scheduled monthly Critical Incident Committee Meetings for the first year of employment.
  - ***Result: Attendance during the reporting period was %.***

Systems-based learning and improvement

- 10 records for Compliance with Anesthesia Care documentation standards according to the compliance program
  - ***Result:***

The following Department of Anesthesiology Chiefs and Medical Directors met to review the Focused Professional Performance Evaluation results on Date of Review. The review was performed by:

- Facility Chief A
- Facility Chief B
- Facility Chief C

Peer review reports that were reviewed for this physician are maintained in the protected peer review files at the Department and/or Medical Staff.

Results of your reviews are attached for your consideration, and we thank you for your attention to this information, and for your contributions in improving the quality of care we provide.

Peer review reports that were reviewed for this physician are maintained in the protected peer review files in the Department and/or the Medical Staff office.

CONFIDENTIAL PROFESSIONAL COMPETENCE/QUALITY REVIEW MATERIAL | DO NOT DUPLICATE OR DISTRIBUTE | CONFIDENTIAL

Fig. 6. The focused professional performance evaluation metrics used currently by the Spectrum Medical Group are shown.

The Joint Commission lists tools available to asses safety culture.[18] Links to available tools to assess safety are provided in the attached references for the following: Safety Attitudes Questionnaire, Agency for Healthcare Research and Quality, and Safety, Communication, Operational Reliability, and Engagement Survey.[19–21]

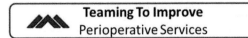

Teaming To Improve
Perioperative Services

Values We Embrace

Patient Centered

- We will focus on the patient at all times; issues are discussed away from the patient care area

Respect

- We will treat each other with respect and fairness in every interaction just as we would want to be treated
- We will recognize and celebrate what each of us contributes to the team
- We will promote courtesy in our interactions, for example, " please", " thank you"

Integrity

- We will raise concerns with each other without assumptions or blame at the right time and right place
- We will be supported at all levels to have open communication when issues arise

Innovation

- We will promote an environment of learning to achieve optimal performance
- We will be open and receptive to new ideas and promote tests of change in our work areas

Excellence

- Anyone on the team will initiate briefings and debriefings; all will participate
- We will introduce ourselves as we would like to be addressed before entering a new work area and include our names on the whiteboard as applicable
- We will anticipate the needs of co-workers
- We will be supported to ask questions when unsure
- We will discuss our common goals and check with our team for any special needs
- We will support perioperative improvement initiatives (ex. OP Z, OP 2.0, OP EX)

Ownership

- We are not above any task that needs to be done
- We will be open about our own frustrations and concerns, for example, stressed, fatigued, or ill
- We will hold ourselves and each other accountable for these tenets

Fig. 7. MMC's current code of conduct, Values We Embrace.

Increasingly the strength of an organization's safety culture is being connected to patient and provider outcomes. Improved safety culture scores have been associated with a reduction in central line–associated blood stream infection and surgical site infection rates.[22,23] Provider Joy in Work is gaining more attention as organizations work to address low provider engagement scores and increasing provider burnout. Joy in Work's connection to health care quality and safety is discussed by the Institute for Healthcare Improvement.[24] In addition, Duke's Patient Safety Center's mission is in part to bring joy back at work, and tools to accomplish this task are discussed (eg, Three Good Things).[25]

When trying to change or strengthen your group's culture, several considerations are provided later. This work is challenging and humbling, as described by James Reason[26]: "It is worth pointing out that if you are convinced that your organization has a good safety culture, you are almost certainly mistaken. Like a state of grace, a safety culture is something that is, striven for but rarely attained. As in religion, the process is more important than the product. The virtue – and the reward – lies in the struggle rather than the outcome."[26]

- Leadership's role: As mentioned in the definition of safety culture earlier and in the references provided, in many ways leadership defines safety culture. Culture starts with leaders.[27]
- Role of an anesthesiologist: All physicians assume a leadership role in each and every OR or procedure room. Anesthesiologists have for too long weakened safety culture by not speaking up when witnessing disrespectful behavior.[28] The importance of leadership, most importantly, how leadership acts on a daily basis, has been discussed previously.
- Recognize that the way that problems are treated reflects your corporate culture.[29]
- Accountability for behaviors: While supporting a blame-free review of human errors and system flaws, disrespectful behavior must not be tolerated. The Maine Medical Center (MMC) has adopted a code of conduct, Values We Embrace **(Fig. 7)**. A clear and consistent process must be in place that fairly addresses the concerns of all caregivers; the consequences must be transparent to all. When disrespectful behavior is addressed effectively, the specifics and results of the investigation are confidential. Team members trust the system's response when they see that the disrespectful behavior ceases. A tool for evaluating an incident is provided in the attached reference.[30]
- Remember everyone needs a voice to feel valued within the organization. The QI committee reinforces this principle when its multidisciplinary membership respects and values the input and concerns from all. Refer to a description of MMC's QI committee provided previously.
- Provide resources and education for individuals to increase their Joy in Work.[25]
- Assess safety culture on a regular basis.[19–21]

SUMMARY

When asked how quality is measured for individual clinicians, there are several principles that guide the answer. Leaders of these individual clinicians must demonstrate daily behaviors that reinforce the group's focus on quality and safety. A strong safety culture that builds trust and encourages an open dialogue about safety concerns, while ensuring that disrespectful or disruptive behavior is not tolerated, will provide a strong foundation for the QMS. Most quality measures reported to individual clinicians will reflect the system's performance. An individual provider should see his or her own data for self-reflection only; these data must not be used for privileging. Finally, data used for privileging (eg, OPPE) must not rely on the QMS and should avoid outcome measures.

REFERENCES

1. Haller G, Stoelwinder J, Myles PS, et al. Quality and safety indicators in anesthesia: a systematic review. Anesthesiology 2009;110(5):1158–75.
2. Motamed C, Bourgain JL. An anaesthesia information management system as a tool for a quality assurance program: 10 years of experience. Anaesth Crit Care Pain Med 2016;35(3):191–5.
3. Naessens JM, Campbell CR, Huddleston JM, et al. A comparison of hospital adverse events identified by three widely used detection methods. Int J Qual Health Care 2009;21(4):301–7.

4. Platz J, Hyman N. Tracking intraoperative complications. J Am Coll Surg 2012; 215(4):519–23.

5. Williams GD, Muffly MK, Mendoza JM, et al. Reporting of perioperative adverse events by pediatric anesthesiologists at a Tertiary Children's Hospital: targeted interventions to increase the rate of reporting. Anesth Analg 2017;125(5): 1515–23.

6. D'Lima DM, Moore J, Bottle A, et al. Developing effective feedback on quality of anaesthetic care: what are its most valuable characteristics from a clinical perspective? J Health Serv Res Policy 2015;20(1 Suppl):26–34.

7. Frenzel JC, Kee SS, Ensor JE, et al. Ongoing provision of individual clinician performance data improves practice behavior. Anesth Analg 2010;111(2):515–9.

8. Glance LG, Hannan EL, Fleisher LA, et al. Feasibility of report cards for measuring anesthesiologist quality for cardiac surgery. Anesth Analg 2016; 122(5):1603–13.

9. Papachristofi O, Mackay JH, Powell SJ, et al. Impact of the anesthesiologist and surgeon on cardiac surgical outcomes. J Cardiothorac Vasc Anesth 2014;28(1): 103–9.

10. Mant J. Process versus outcome indicators in the assessment of quality of health care. Int J Qual Health Care 2001;13(6):475–80.

11. Krell RW, Hozain A, Kao LS, et al. Reliability of risk-adjusted outcomes for profiling hospital surgical quality. JAMA Surg 2014;149(5):467–74.

12. Rhoads KF, Wren SM. Understanding the reliability of American College of Surgeons National Surgical Quality Improvement Program as a quality comparator. JAMA Surg 2014;149(5):474.

13. Kohn LT, Corrigan J, Donaldson MS. To err is human: building a safer health system. Washington, DC: National Academy Press; 2000.

14. Deming WE. Out of the crisis. 1st edition. Cambridge (MA): MIT Press; 2000.

15. Commission TJ. Ongoing professional practice evaluation (OPPE)- intent. 2017. Available at: https://www.jointcommission.org/standards_information/jcfaqdetails. aspx?StandardsFaqId=1431&ProgramId=46. Accessed October 4, 2017.

16. National Civil Aviation Review Commission. Avoiding aviation gridlock & reducing the accident rate: a consensus for change. Washington, DC: National Civil Aviation Review Commission; 1997.

17. Moscucci M, Eagle KA, Share D, et al. Public reporting and case selection for percutaneous coronary interventions: an analysis from two large multicenter percutaneous coronary intervention databases. J Am Coll Cardiol 2005;45(11):1759–65.

18. The Joint Commission, USA. The essential role of leadership in developing a safety culture. Sentinel Event Alert 2017;(57):1–8.

19. Sexton JB, Helmreich RL, Neilands TB, et al. The safety attitudes questionnaire: psychometric properties, benchmarking data, and emerging research. BMC Health Serv Res 2006;6:44.

20. Safe & Reliable Healthcare L. SCORE: survey of safety, communication, organizational reliability, resilience/burnout and engagement. 2017. Available at: https://www.safeandreliablecare.com/surveys/. Accessed October 9, 2017.

21. Quality AfHRa. Surveys on patient safety culture. 2012. Available at: https://www. ahrq.gov/professionals/quality-patient-safety/patientsafetyculture/index.html. Accessed October 9, 2017.

22. Sagana R, Hyzy RC. Achieving zero central line-associated bloodstream infection rates in your intensive care unit. Crit Care Clin 2013;29(1):1–9.

23. Fan CJ, Pawlik TM, Daniels T, et al. Association of safety culture with surgical site infection outcomes. J Am Coll Surg 2016;222(2):122–8.

24. Institute for Healthcare Improvement. Joy in work. 2017. Available at: http://www.ihi.org/Topics/Joy-In-Work/Pages/default.aspx. Accessed October 9, 2017.

25. Center DPS. Training, research and implementation for patient safety and quality. 2017. Available at: http://www.dukepatientsafetycenter.com/. Accessed October 9, 2017.

26. Reason JT. Managing the risks of organizational accidents. Aldershot (United Kingdom): Ashgate; 1997.

27. Brashears L. Culture is a business issue. Venture Capital Review 2012;(28): 55–60.

28. Anesthesia Quality Institute. A case report from the anesthesia incident reporting system. ASA Monitor 2016;80(10):50–3.

29. Shook J. How to change a culture: lessons from NUMMI. MIT Sloan Manag Rev 2010;51(2):63.

30. Chassin MR. Building your safety culture: a job for leaders. 2017. Available at: https://www.jointcommission.org/assets/1/6/webinar_replay_sea_57_slides.pdf. Accessed October 9, 2017.

Challenges in Outcome Reporting

Avery Tung, MD

KEYWORDS

- Outcome reporting • Risk adjustment • Quality improvement

KEY POINTS

- Challenges with outcome reporting include definition, measurement, and risk adjustment.
- Outcome reporting programs may have unintended consequences, including clinician reluctance to care for high-risk patients.
- Neither effective risk adjustment nor precise measurement is needed to improve care.

INTRODUCTION

Since the publication of the 1999 Institute of Medicine's report on medical error,[1] organized medicine has struggled to apply quality improvement principles from nonmedical domains to patient care. Among these principles are a belief that variability in the delivery of care must represent unwarranted deviation from optimal care, that physicians should change behavior to minimize such deviation, and that comparing physicians based on process or outcome ultimately results in better care.

Although such principles sound plausible, their real world performance is surprisingly uneven. Almost 30 years ago, Donabedian[2] first published his taxonomy of quality measurement,[2] categorizing medical quality as either structure, process, or outcome based. As examples, structural aspects of quality might include nurse/patient ratios, presence of rapid response teams, and/or specialized intensive care unit (ICU) staffing. Process-related quality involves technical aspects of clinical care: how often beta-blockers are given, whether glucose levels are kept within specific boundaries, or whether formal handoffs between providers are performed. Outcome-related quality involves measurement of the result of medical care and includes the incidence of end points, such as renal failure, reintubation, or surgical site infections.

Although remembered today as a strong advocate for medical quality improvement, Donabedian[2] expressed considerable skepticism in his landmark article regarding

Disclosures: This article was not supported by any external funding sources. Dr A. Tung receives a salary as executive editor for *Critical Care and Resuscitation, Anesthesia & Analgesia.*
Department of Anesthesia and Critical Care, University of Chicago, 5841 South Maryland Avenue MC 4028, Chicago, IL 60637, USA
E-mail address: atung@dacc.uchicago.edu

Anesthesiology Clin 36 (2018) 191–199
https://doi.org/10.1016/j.anclin.2018.01.004
1932-2275/18/© 2018 Elsevier Inc. All rights reserved.

how well his 3 categories of quality mapped to true quality of care. Donabedian[2] described the relationship between structural aspects of medical care and the process of care as "rather weak," observed that our knowledge regarding the relationship between technical care and outcome is of dubious quality and that assessments of the quality of technical care may vary, and doubted strongly that "direct assessment of the outcome of care can free us from imperfections of clinical science."[2]

The recently concluded 8-year experiment in surgical process measurement, the infamous Surgical Care Improvement Project (SCIP) program, suggests that although process measurement clearly improves adherence to the measured processes, outcomes may not improve. Despite targeted processes being evidence based, no perioperative SCIP measure has to date consistently improved its associated outcome. This finding is even true for interventions with extensive pre-SCIP literature support, such as subcutaneous heparin for deep venous thrombosis prophylaxis.[3] In light of such poor efficacy, and the quiet retirement of the SCIP program in January 2015, policymakers have worried that the forced measurement and reporting of process measures may not be the most effective use of limited quality resources.

The realization that process improvement may not lead to outcome improvement also suggests that an alternate strategy of measuring outcomes may be more effective. Conceptually, outcome measurement may improve quality by 2 mechanisms. The first is that outcome measurement forces physicians to examine their outcomes and in doing so helps them to identify potential quality issues. The second is that outcome measurement identifies physicians or practices with particularly good outcomes. By studying practices with good outcomes, physicians can then incrementally move toward better processes and (it is hoped) better outcomes.

Unfortunately, outcome reporting introduces its own set of challenges. Among these are difficulties in defining an outcome, identifying appropriate benchmarks, effective risk adjustment, gaming, the importance of definition, and unintended consequences, including care for high-risk, high-acuity patients. This article briefly describes these challenges and suggests strategies for effectively harnessing outcome reporting for improving anesthesia quality.

WHAT IS AN OUTCOME AND WHAT IS A GOOD OUTCOME?

Unlike process measures, which are easily described, outcomes can often be surprisingly difficult to define and measure. For example, 3 popular definitions of acute kidney injury (AKI) exist: the National Surgical Improvement Project (NSQIP), Acute Kidney Injury Network (AKIN), and Risk Injury and Failure and Loss and End stage kidney disease (RIFLE) criteria. The NSQIP definition is triggered when serum creatinine exceeds 2 mmol/dL or when dialysis is initiated, whereas the AKIN and RIFLE criteria are not based on dialysis, involve urine output metrics, and include relative increases in creatinine from baseline.[4] It is easy to see, and studies have demonstrated,[5] that the more rigorous NSQIP criteria underestimate the incidence of milder forms of AKI.

Other clinically relevant outcomes, such as stroke, are similarly troublesome. The Society for Neuroscience in Anesthesiology and Critical Care defines stroke as a brain infarction of ischemic or hemorrhagic cause that occurs during or within 30 days of surgery.[6] Although this definition is straightforward, if a focal deficit is clearly expressed and a corresponding brain lesion is visible on imaging, or if the computed tomography scan is negative, or the symptoms are not clearly focal, or patients recovers partial or full function within 2 or 3 weeks, then should the condition really be declared a stroke? Such judgments can require a disturbing level of subjectivity.

The *treated normal* condition also muddies the waters with respect to outcome definition. The *International Classification of Diseases, Tenth Revision's* definition of cardiogenic shock (R57.0), for example, is defined as "a life-threatening medical condition resulting from an inadequate circulation of blood due to primary failure of the ventricles of the heart to function effectively." But if patients are effectively supported by multiple pressors/inotropes or an assist device, such as a left ventricular assist device or balloon pump, then are patients still in shock? Reasonable people may disagree, with some arguing that the presence of an assist device or inotrope administration automatically activates a diagnosis of cardiogenic shock and others requiring an elevated lactate or creatinine level. Similar questions might be asked of patients with hypothyroid receiving adequate medication or normotensive patients receiving antihypertensive medications. If they exhibit no symptoms of their disease while receiving medication, then arguably they do not meet criteria for the disease.

Another current example is the Agency for Healthcare Research and Quality patient safety indicator 11 (PSI-11) (postoperative respiratory failure). This metric takes on greater significance in 2017, as it now comprises 30% of the PSI-90 composite perioperative quality metric. PSI-11 is triggered when patients are reintubated anytime during their postoperative hospital stay, a diagnosis of postoperative respiratory failure is entered into the record, or if they leave the operating room intubated but cannot be extubated within 96 hours.

Although such an outcome seems easy to define, anesthesiologists may often choose to leave patients intubated postoperatively as a precaution in patients at risk for large fluid shifts, difficult-to-control pain, or airway management concerns.[7] Such patients present coding dilemmas, as they are only intubated for prophylactic reasons (and, thus, do not have postoperative respiratory failure per se). Coding them as *postoperative respiratory failure* (J95.821) triggers the metric, whereas coding them as *acute pulmonary insufficiency following surgery* (J95.2) does not. Clearly, reasonable caregivers may disagree as to the specific diagnosis.

Taken together, these examples suggest that defining an outcome, although easy in principle, can often become considerably more difficult when the complexity of perioperative care is considered. To further compound the challenge of outcome definition, identifying a benchmark for measurement can also be difficult. Published rates of ICU delirium may vary from 11%[8] to 80%,[9] and mortality with acute respiratory distress syndrome may vary from 25% to 58%.[10,11] Even the incidence of AKI after abdominal surgery may vary more than 15-fold.[12] In light of such variability, merely determining whether the incidence of the measured outcome represents quality care may not be straightforward.

RISK ADJUSTMENT: PROBLEM OR SOLUTION?

In principle, some of the variability in benchmark outcomes described earlier may be erased by adjusting for known comorbidities and other factors that may affect outcomes. Patients with preexisting renal insufficiency are more prone to postoperative AKI,[13] and those with preoperative dementia have a higher incidence of postoperative delirium.[14] By adjusting for such preexisting conditions, physicians from different practices may more easily compare outcomes.

In practice, however, effective risk adjustment is extremely difficult. Multiple older studies have demonstrated that risk-adjustment algorithms often fail to agree with each other,[15,16] and modern attempts to compare hospitals using different risk-adjustment algorithms have performed poorly in ranking hospitals by mortality rate.[17] Such studies consistently find that hospitals rated poorly using one risk-adjustment paradigm may be rated highly using another paradigm, suggesting that the choice of risk-adjustment system plays an important role. Even risk-adjusted mortality rates for a single operation, aortic valve replacement for stenosis, may vary by almost 2-fold in their predictions,[18] and ranking cardiac surgery programs by risk-adjusted mortality can lead to wild swings in year-to-year rankings.[19] Taken together, these findings suggest that adjusting for severity of patient illness may not level the playing field as much as might be imagined.

Worse yet, risk adjustment may induce gaming behavior, as physicians act to optimize their public performance reports. The introduction of risk-adjusted report cards for cardiac surgeons in New York State was followed by 7-fold increases in the incidence of renal failure, 3-fold increases in the incidence of chronic obstructive pulmonary disease, and 4-fold increases in the incidence of congestive heart failure.[20] Although such increases are theoretically possible, a more likely explanation is that physicians rapidly identified which factors were used in risk adjustment and began coding those conditions more aggressively. When viewed in light of the *treated normal* problem described earlier, human nature suggests that to maximize their risk-adjusted mortality, physicians may move to, for example, assign a diagnosis of cardiogenic shock to patients receiving dobutamine even if blood pressure, lactate levels, and renal function are all normal.

Existing real-world experience suggests that successful gaming behavior may easily track ahead of risk-adjustment efforts. The introduction of risk adjustment into per-person payments for the Medicare Advantage insurance program in 2004 was originally intended to permit Medicare to better predict medical costs. Whereas before risk-adjustment payments were adjusted only for demographic factors, the 2004 update introduced a series of patient conditions to enhance risk adjustment.[21] Although the predictive effect of the model increased, payments also increased, as private managers realized that more parameters allowed more aggressive coding and that identifying healthy patients within a certain condition category could be extremely lucrative. Offering fitness memberships to patients for switching to Medicare Advantage is an example of a successful attempt to attract a healthier patient population.[22] Liberally coding such patients for associated disease conditions then allows insurance companies to bill for high-severity conditions while caring for relatively healthy patients. In fact, data suggest that such favorable risk selection may not have decreased with the introduction of more rigorous risk adjustment.[23]

THE EFFECT OF DEFINITION ON THE INDIVIDUAL PROVIDER

As noted earlier, defining an outcome can be difficult. But even if an outcome can be unambiguously defined, small changes can significantly affect individual providers because of baseline differences in patient populations. As an example, at the University of Chicago, 30-day postoperative AKI rates range from 3% to 4%; but considerable variability exists among individual providers. However, varying the time window from 3 to 60 days not only changes the overall incidence of postoperative AKI (as expected) but also changes the relative rank of individual providers within the department. Providers may change relative rank by as much as 50%, easily enough to transform some from best to worst performers. This effect occurs because the trajectory of postoperative AKI differs among different patient classes; providers caring for vascular surgery patients, for example, have a high long-term risk of AKI but a relatively small short-term risk. In contrast, patients undergoing cardiopulmonary bypass may have a higher short-term risk but a smaller long-term risk. A short window for perioperative AKI may then favor one type of patient over others.

Such a difference renders adequate risk adjustment even more difficult, as subtle differences between patients in their long-term postoperative course can meaningfully affect individual provider ranks and unfairly penalize some providers while rewarding others.

UNINTENDED CONSEQUENCES

Ideally, a provider receiving feedback on his or her outcomes and provided with risk-adjusted comparisons with his or her peers would focus on improving aspects of care that may meaningfully affect outcomes. But, as Donabedian observed, linkages between processes of care and outcomes are discouragingly weak. The recently concluded SCIP, which mandated public reporting of perioperative process measure adherence, indicates that Donabedian's observations have held up with time. SCIP data suggest, disconcertingly, that antibiotic administration within 1 hour of surgery has a limited effect on perioperative surgical site infection[24] and that perioperative venous thromboembolism prophylaxis[3,25] is poorly correlated to venous thromboembolism rates.

The strongest predictors of perioperative outcomes remain preoperative patient comorbidities. In studies of AKI, for example, intraoperative factors, such as vasoconstrictor use, have only a modest effect on predictive models based on preoperative data.[26] A rational reaction to comparative outcome measurement might then be to avoid caring for sicker patients and, thus, adversely affecting one's outcomes. Such behavior has been documented previously with the outmigration of cardiac surgery patients from New York,[27] reduced access to cardiac surgery for minorities likely to be high risk,[28] and reluctance to undertake high-risk percutaneous coronary intervention (PCI) in states with public outcome reporting.[29] One 2012 study found that the introduction of public reporting of PCI outcomes in Boston reduced the use of PCI in cardiogenic shock by almost 25% when compared with states without public reporting.[30]

Although risk adjustment in principle can mitigate the outcome penalty incurred by physicians working with high-risk patients, studies in nonmedical domains suggest that evaluators use risk adjustment only minimally in judging performance. A 2013 study from the University of California and Harvard business schools found that master of business administration admissions officers were more likely to accept students with high grade point averages even when told that their schools had lax grading standards.[31] The argument that risk adjustment effectively places physicians on a level playing field may, thus, not convince health care users that a hospital with higher mortality rates is, nevertheless, equivalent or better than its competitor because it cares for sicker patients.

OUTCOME REPORTING HAS INTRINSIC VALUE

Despite the myriad flaws in outcome reporting, it has intrinsic value and should be an integral part of anesthesia quality management. An important challenge in anesthesia quality is acquiring feedback about outcomes that occur outside the immediate postoperative period. Outcomes, such as AKI, death, sepsis, myocardial infarction, and stroke, rarely occur on postoperative day 0, which requires the anesthesiologist to somehow track patients after they leave the postoperative care unit.

Without such feedback, however, modifying anesthetic practice is considerably more difficult. Anesthesiologists make multiple perioperative decisions in the face of uncertainty: to cancel a case, treat an elevated glucose or thyroid-stimulating hormone level, transfuse, beta block, or target a mean pressure; the consequences of such decisions may not manifest until later. Without knowing those consequences, optimizing intraoperative decision-making may take considerably longer.

Arguments that risk adjustment is flawed and prevents fair comparisons between practitioners are valid. But such comparisons are not needed to improve quality. Physicians can always strive to get better by individual case review, thoughtful analysis, iterative changes, and ongoing monitoring. Viewed cynically, risk adjustment either leads to complacency for caregivers with apparently sicker-than-average patients or distrust in caregivers with apparently less sick patients. Ideally caregivers should strive for no adverse events, rather than accept a nonzero risk-adjusted rate that makes them better than average. The history of cardiac surgery suggests that this incremental approach may lead to dramatic improvements in outcomes, as clinicians rapidly progressed from early attempts with 50% mortality[32] to calls for a 1% 30-day mortality rate for coronary artery bypass grafting procedures.[33] Improvements in extracorporeal membrane oxygenation[34] outcomes have largely occurred using the same incremental process.

The assertion that difficulty in precisely defining and measuring outcomes prevents clinicians from improving quality is similarly misplaced. An oft-heard tenet of organized medical quality is the American industrialist William Deming's[35] assertion that "if you can't measure it, you can't improve it." But this quote takes Deming's point out of context. His actual quote reads "It is wrong to suppose that if you can't measure it you can't manage it – a costly myth."[35] In fact, Deming noted that many critically important figures in manufacturing or production 'are unknown or unknowable, but successful management must nevertheless take account of them.[35]

After some consideration, Deming's argument that even complex, difficult-to-measure attributes can be managed successfully becomes reasonable. TV makeovers clearly demonstrate that making oneself better looking is possible, even if consensus metrics on beauty are not available. Arguably, the task of improving the most important perioperative outcomes is sufficiently complex that the most efficient way forward is incremental, feedback-based improvement.

SUMMARY

Thirty years after Donabedian's classification of medical quality improvement into structure, process, and outcome focused, policymakers have come to appreciate his concern that efforts to improve structural or process measures often fail to improve their associated outcomes. By turning to comparative outcome measurement as a tool for improving quality, quality strategists are implying that targeted, specific process improvement may not effectively improve outcomes and suggesting that individual efforts to improve outcomes may yield results more rapidly.

Efforts to accelerate that process by comparing outcomes among hospitals and providers, however, have introduced a series of complications. Among them are complexities in generating universally accepted definitions and how outcomes are to be identified. Although cheapest, monitoring strategies based on administrative or billing solutions rely on coding consistency, which may vary widely from one hospital and provider to another. The *treated normal* condition, whereby patients have a known condition but are clinically normal because of treatment, presents a particular challenge in perioperative care. Whether patients receiving dobutamine after cardiac surgery with normal serum lactate levels have cardiogenic shock, for example, is an open question. An example of how a treated state may be interpreted differently as a consequence of an outcome measure is the PSI-11 quality indicator, *postoperative respiratory failure*. Whether patients intubated after surgery for airway protection, pain management, or hypothermia should be included in this metric is unclear.

For nearly all comparative outcome reporting, risk adjustment is considered necessary to account for patient mix or disease severity. However, although individual risk-adjustment models may themselves predict outcomes effectively, they may not be consistent from one data set to another and may not rank providers the same way. This variability in ranking limits the use of risk-adjustment tools in large-scale quality programs, as disagreement regarding the appropriate adjustment tool may prevent widespread acceptance. By introducing more variables into a provider score, complex risk-adjustment protocols may also invite gaming behavior.

Outcome reporting may induce other unintended consequences. The most concerning potential consequence is the tendency of clinicians to avoid caring for patients at high risk for a bad outcome. Evidence that such behavior occurs as a consequence of public reporting exists in the New York State cardiac surgery database and in public reporting programs for PCI in Massachusetts. Such a behavior may exacerbate health care disparities by denying care to underserved patients at higher likelihood for poor outcomes.

However, ultimately outcome reporting is a vital element of the quality manager's toolbox. In light of poor relationships between process and structural metrics of quality and actual outcomes, an advantage of outcome reporting is that it allows greater leeway for individual hospitals and providers to identify practices that optimize outcomes. Particularly for anesthesiologists who may not participate in patients' care beyond the first postoperative day, outcome reporting provides valuable feedback without which the ability to refine perioperative clinical decision-making is limited.

Although risk adjustment may be imperfect, clinicians need not compare themselves with others to improve. Individual case review, incremental adjustment, and identification of good and bad practices can be extremely effective; such practices should be an aspect of every clinician's quality-improvement approach. Finally, an inability to precisely quantitate an outcome or process should likewise not deter clinicians from striving to improve. As Deming noted, many processes cannot be precisely measured, yet must be managed, and often are successfully. Ultimately, outcome reporting has the potential to lead to considerable improvements in care and should be considered an integral part of every anesthesiologist's quality program.

REFERENCES

1. Institute of Medicine. To err is human: building a safer health system. Washington, DC: The National Academies Press; 2000.
2. Donabedian A. The quality of care. How can it be assessed? JAMA 1988;260(12): 1743–8.
3. Johnbull EA, Lau BD, Schneider EB, et al. No association between hospital-reported perioperative venous thromboembolism prophylaxis and outcome rates in publicly reported data. JAMA Surg 2014;149(4):400–1.
4. Chang CH, Lin CY, Tian YC, et al. Acute kidney injury classification: comparison of AKIN and RIFLE criteria. Shock 2010;33(3):247–52.
5. Bihorac A, Brennan M, Ozrazgat-Baslanti T, et al. National surgical quality improvement program underestimates the risk associated with mild and moderate postoperative acute kidney injury. Crit Care Med 2013;41(11): 2570–83.
6. Mashour GA, Moore LE, Lele AV, et al. Perioperative care of patients at high risk for stroke during or after non-cardiac, non-neurologic surgery: consensus

statement from the Society for Neuroscience in Anesthesiology and Critical Care. J Neurosurg Anesthesiol 2014;26(4):273–85.

7. Ray JJ, Degnan M, Rao KA, et al. Incidence and operative factors associated with discretional postoperative mechanical ventilation after general surgery. Anesth Analg 2018;126(2):489–94.

8. Aldemir M, Ozen S, Kara IH, et al. Predisposing factors for delirium in the surgical intensive care unit. Crit Care 2001;5(5):265–70.

9. Ely EW, Shintani A, Truman B, et al. Delirium as a predictor of mortality in mechanically ventilated patients in the intensive care unit. JAMA 2004;291(14):1753–62.

10. Brower RG, Lanken PN, MacIntyre N, et al, National Heart, Lung, and Blood Institute ARDS Clinical Trials Network. Higher versus lower positive end-expiratory pressures in patients with the acute respiratory distress syndrome. N Engl J Med 2004;351(4):327–36.

11. Estenssoro E, Dubin A, Laffaire E, et al. Incidence, clinical course, and outcome in 217 patients with acute respiratory distress syndrome. Crit Care Med 2002; 30(11):2450–6.

12. Kim M, Brady JE, Li G. Variations in the risk of acute kidney injury across intraabdominal surgery procedures. Anesth Analg 2014;119(5):1121–32.

13. Kheterpal S, Tremper KK, Heung M, et al. Development and validation of an acute kidney injury risk index for patients undergoing general surgery: results from a national data set. Anesthesiology 2009;110(3):505–15.

14. Lee HB, Mears SC, Rosenberg PB, et al. Predisposing factors for postoperative delirium after hip fracture repair in individuals with and without dementia. J Am Geriatr Soc 2011;59(12):2306–13.

15. Iezzoni LI. The risks of risk adjustment. JAMA 1997;278(19):1600–7.

16. Iezzoni LI, Ash AS, Shwartz M, et al. Predicting in-hospital deaths from coronary artery bypass graft surgery. Do different severity measures give different predictions? Med Care 1998;36(1):28–39.

17. Shahian DM, Wolf RE, Iezzoni LI, et al. Variability in the measurement of hospital-wide mortality rates. N Engl J Med 2010;363(26):2530–9.

18. Yamaoka H, Kuwaki K, Inaba H, et al. Comparison of modern risk scores in predicting operative mortality for patients undergoing aortic valve replacement for aortic stenosis. J Cardiol 2016;68(2):135–40.

19. Siregar S, Groenwold RH, Jansen EK, et al. Limitations of ranking lists based on cardiac surgery mortality rates. Circ Cardiovasc Qual Outcomes 2012;5(3): 403–9.

20. Green J, Wintfeld N. Report cards on cardiac surgeons. Assessing New York State's approach. N Engl J Med 1995;332(18):1229–32.

21. Pope GC, Kautter J, Ellis RP, et al. Risk adjustment of Medicare capitation payments using the CMS-HCC model. Health Care Financ Rev 2004;25(4):119–41.

22. Cooper AL, Trivedi AN. Fitness memberships and favorable selection in Medicare Advantage plans. N Engl J Med 2012;366(2):150–7.

23. Goldberg EM, Trivedi AN, Mor V, et al. Favorable risk selection in Medicare advantage: trends in mortality and plan exits among nursing home beneficiaries. Med Care Res Rev 2017;74(6):736–49.

24. Hawn MT, Richman JS, Vick CC, et al. Timing of surgical antibiotic prophylaxis and the risk of surgical site infection. JAMA Surg 2013;148(7):649–57.

25. Altom LK, Deierhoi RJ, Grams J, et al. Association between Surgical Care Improvement Program venous thromboembolism measures and postoperative events. Am J Surg 2012;204(5):591–7.

26. Kheterpal S, Tremper KK, Englesbe MJ, et al. Predictors of postoperative acute renal failure after noncardiac surgery in patients with previously normal renal function. Anesthesiology 2007;107(6):892–902.
27. Omoigui NA, Miller DP, Brown KJ, et al. Outmigration for coronary bypass surgery in an era of public dissemination of clinical outcomes. Circulation 1996;93(1): 27–33.
28. Werner RM, Asch DA, Polsky D. Racial profiling: the unintended consequences of coronary artery bypass graft report cards. Circulation 2005;111(10):1257–63.
29. Moscucci M, Eagle KA, Share D, et al. Public reporting and case selection for percutaneous coronary interventions: an analysis from two large multicenter percutaneous coronary intervention databases. J Am Coll Cardiol 2005;45(11): 1759–65.
30. Joynt KE, Blumenthal DM, Orav EJ, et al. Association of public reporting for percutaneous coronary intervention with utilization and outcomes among Medicare beneficiaries with acute myocardial infarction. JAMA 2012;308(14):1460–8.
31. Swift SA, Moore DA, Sharek ZS, et al. Inflated applicants: attribution errors in performance evaluation by professionals. PLoS One 2013;8(7):e69258.
32. Kirklin JW, Dushane JW, Patrick RT, et al. Intracardiac surgery with the aid of a mechanical pump-oxygenator system (gibbon type): report of eight cases. Proc Staff Meet Mayo Clin 1955;30(10):201–6.
33. Mack MJ. If this were my last speech, what would I say? Ann Thorac Surg 2012; 94(4):1044–52.
34. Thiagarajan RR, Barbaro RP, Rycus PT, et al, ELSO Member Centers. Extracorporeal Life Support Organization Registry International report 2016. ASAIO J 2017; 63(1):60–7.
35. Deming WE. The new economics: for industry, government, education. 2nd edition. Cambridge (MA): MIT Press; 2000.

Quality Reporting
Understanding National Priorities, Identifying Local Applicability

DeLaine Schmitz, MSHL, RN[a], Matthew T. Popovich, PhD[b],*

KEYWORDS

- Anesthesia • Registry • Quality • Measurement • Feasibility • NACOR • CMS
- NQF

KEY POINTS

- When considering quality measures to collect and report, practices should understand the larger framework and priorities of payers and the healthcare community.
- Practices may develop and use local quality improvement measures based on local needs but measures used for quality reporting by national entities and payers must undergo a more rigorous and well-defined process.
- Anesthesia practices face a significant amount of challenges when reporting data to a registry, most significantly when merging data files from multiple data sources.
- Practice champions and practice leadership should explore how registry reporting can be used for meeting federal reporting requirements and improving patient care locally.

Since the 1990s, the use of quality measures among a variety of healthcare stakeholders has grown at an exponential rate. Practices must not only maintain current knowledge of the measures that affect individual physicians and other clinicians locally but also understand how the assessment of these medical professionals by such quality measures may affect the priorities and quality activities of facility administration staff. Moreover, because quality measures are increasingly used by hospital administrators, health plans, and payers, practices must contemplate whether the

Disclosure Statement: The American Society of Anesthesiologists (ASA) and its affiliate Anesthesia Quality Institute (AQI) operate the National Anesthesia Clinical Outcomes Registry (NACOR). AQI NACOR is a Patient Safety Organization as well as a Qualified Registry and Qualified Clinical Data Registry that practices may use to submit data to federal reporting programs. AQI NACOR is an ASA member benefit. Non-ASA members must pay a fee for using AQI NACOR.
[a] American Society of Anesthesiologists, 1061 American Lane, Schaumburg, IL 60173, USA;
[b] American Society of Anesthesiologists, 905 16th Street Northwest, Suite 400, Washington, DC 20006, USA
* Corresponding author.
E-mail address: M.Popovich@asahq.org

Anesthesiology Clin 36 (2018) 201–216
https://doi.org/10.1016/j.anclin.2018.01.009   anesthesiology.theclinics.com
1932-2275/18/© 2018 Elsevier Inc. All rights reserved.

measures they choose to report are common among their peers and are objective. They must also have the ability to differentiate their care from other practices and clinicians. Although it may seem like a dog-eat-dog world, competitiveness and quantifying differences is unfortunately the framework that practices encounter today.

Practices are often compelled to report quality measures based on external factors. For measures incorporated in federal payment programs, for instance, those measures used in the Physician Quality Reporting System (PQRS) (2007–2016) and its successor, the Merit-Based Incentive Payment System (MIPS) Quality Component, public and private payers will require that the quality measures undergo a rigorous development process that follows standard measure development processes.[1] Accreditation organizations may also require practices to collect and report quality measures as part of an accreditation requirement or quality assurance and performance improvement activity.[2]

In other cases, practices may include their reporting of quality measures and performance improvement activities within contracts they hold with the hospital or facilities where they work. When practices are responsible for federal quality reporting themselves (outside of the hospital quality administration), hospital administrators may include certain reporting requirements for the practice to meet. In other cases, contracts may require that the practice identify measures or metrics to collect and report to the administration. Performance on these measures is often tied to payment bonuses or incentives.

Regardless of whether a practice chooses to voluntarily report or feels compelled to report a measure, the process of quality measure development, quality reporting, and gathering quality feedback reports relies significantly on transparency. Transparency in the quality reporting process also works to improve buy-in from clinicians and the processes used for identifying when and where process improvements should take place. Yet, at the same time, transparency does not suggest that every practice will understand measure algorithms, reliability, validity, or a measure's significance to clinical care. Transparency likewise does not mean that patients or caregivers will be able to use that data to make rational choices when choosing a physician or practice.

UNDERSTANDING MEASURE INFLUENCERS

When considering quality measures to collect and report, practices should understand the larger framework and priorities of payers and the healthcare community. Federal legislation requires the Centers for Medicare & Medicaid Services (CMS) to annually publish and update its Measure Development Plan (MDP). The MDP "provides a foundation for building a measure portfolio for the Quality Payment Program and identifies initial priorities among clinical specialties, quality domains, and measurement gaps."[3] After more than 2 decades of quality measure development, often without a united or coherent strategy, the CMS has been given considerable influence over measure development and direction.

The most recent MDP deemphasized measures that practices and clinicians often consider as process, attestation, or check-box measures. Although these measures are expected to be available for reporting in the short term, the trend away from measures such as the administration of prophylactic antibiotic or use of an interoperative warming device has already begun.[4] Replacement of these measures has become most urgent among measure developers as the CMS and payers emphasize other measures considered as high-priority. High priority measures include those process measures that have a direct impact to patient outcomes, care coordination, and patient satisfaction.

Additional attention from payers, developers, and other healthcare stakeholders has focused on the use of electronic resources. Electronic data can be used to verify that precise actions or patient outcomes have been accurately captured for measure reporting. Whereas some process measures can be captured by attestation (eg, via a check box), electronic Clinical Quality Measures are likely to include a more comprehensive documentation trail that a clinical action or outcome occurred.

In recent years, the CMS has collaborated with the American Health Insurance Plans to determine common measures for certain specialists to report. Known as the Core Quality Measures Collaborative, the actions of this group resulted in a common set of quality measures for some, but not all, specialties.[5] Anesthesiology, a specialty with arguably a smaller measure set than most others, was left out of these preliminary discussions. Without a common direction from the CMS or even private insurers, anesthesia practices were, on 1 hand, left without a clear set of measures that could be reported across multiple payers and care settings but, on the other hand, were allowed more flexibility to choose the measures that most affected their practice.

The public–private discussions of the Core Quality Measures Collaborative represented just 1 element of communication between physicians, clinicians, payers, hospital administrations, health insurance companies, Medicaid administrators, and other healthcare stakeholders on quality reporting. The challenge of facilitating communication between these stakeholders has long been recognized. However, in the early 2000s, the National Quality Forum (NQF) emerged as a major force in implementing a consensus-based process for measure evaluation and endorsement.[6] The NQF receives funding from the federal government yet was established as a public–private membership organization composed of a variety of stakeholders. Membership dues account for about one-third of their funding.[7] In its evaluation of quality measures, the NQF solicits experts from their membership to review and assess quality measures based on objective criteria. Measure endorsement requires a public comment period, as well as a vote by NQF members.[8] An NQF decision on a measure can lead CMS and other payers to adopt the measure in varying payment programs.

Practices should consider their medical associations as influencers in measure development and use. Medical associations, first lead by the American Medical Association Physician Consortium for Performance Improvement in the 2000s and later joined by individual medical associations such as the American Society of Anesthesiologists (ASA), the American College of Surgeons, and the Society of Thoracic Surgeons (STS) contribute extensively to the measurement community. The CMS and other payers often look to medical societies to develop measures that are meaningful to their members and specialty. The CMS routinely engages medical associations on applicable quality measures to use in payment programs. Societies that have robust medical registries also look to their members to learn which measures are most meaningful, applicable, and feasible to report.

KEY COMPONENTS OF MEASURE DEVELOPMENT

Quality reporting depends on a robust, defensible, and meaningful measure development process. Although practices may wish to identify local quality improvement measures based on specific patient populations and interventions, measures used for quality reporting by national entities and payers must undergo a more rigorous and well-defined process. The measure development process is defined by both the CMS and the NQF. Each year, the CMS updates and publishes its Measure Management System Blueprint, a document that assists CMS contractors and measure developers on the proper ways to develop quality measures.[1] Within this process, a measure developer relies on clinical experts, patients, and other stakeholders to build and test a measure (**Figs. 1** and **2**).

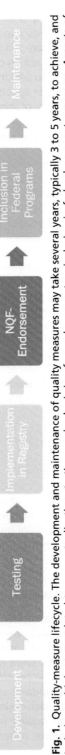

Fig. 1. Quality-measure lifecycle. The development and maintenance of quality measures may take several years, typically 3 to 5 years, to achieve, and includes multiple steps related to conceptualization, testing, and submission for endorsement or inclusion in federal payment programs. Aspects of measure development that depend on stakeholders outside of the measure developer or steward are included.

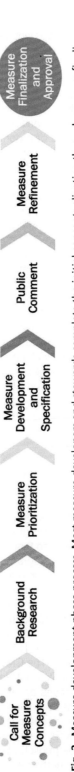

Fig. 2. Measure development phase process. Most measure developers and stewards complete the initial conceptualization through measure finalization based on expert opinion, testing, and public comment periods. The individual processes within the first step of the quality measure lifecycle are reflected.

Of the many processes of measure development, there are a few key components that practices should understand. Physician experts, methodologists, statisticians, informaticists, clinical subject matter experts, and other stakeholders, such as patients, are often gathered by the developer to form a technical expert panel (TEP). A TEP manages and influences which measure concepts will eventually become quality measures. Building the measure from a concept takes time, patience, and constructive discussions to hone the measure's intent, collection method, and usability at the individual clinician level.

A quality measure, at its core, consists of a denominator and numerator. The denominator is a statement that describes the population evaluated by the quality measure. Denominators often include Current Procedural Terminology (CPT) Codes, *International Statistical Classification of Diseases and Related Health Problems*, 10th revision, codes, or other patient population elements, such as age, diagnosis or condition, and anesthesia type. Measure stewards must be careful in crafting the denominator as a measure. They should only include those patients for whom the clinical action or outcome is chosen to be measured. The measure numerator is a statement of the measure's target process, procedure, clinical action, or outcome.

Measure TEPs must also consider if any patients or actions should be excluded from the measure's performance. Denominator exclusions and exceptions are often used to hone and narrow the measure when appropriate. Denominator exclusions are patients who should be removed from the measure population and denominator before determining if numerator criteria are met. Denominator exceptions allow for an adjustment of the calculated score. Exceptions allow for the exercise of clinical judgment and are most often used for medical reasons (eg, allergic to certain intervention), patient reasons (eg, lack of communication), or system reasons.[1] In each of these cases, practices should record and report the specific exclusion and exception codes to the registry or the CMS.

As the measure approaches its final phases, measure developers will launch a public comment period. The public comment period is used to gather constructive feedback and identify any concerns or problems that practices, clinicians, or patients may see with the construction and potential use of a measure. The CMS and other measure developers, including specialty societies, provide for public comment periods. At this point in the process, practices may wish to provide expert comment on how they may use the measure, any problems a practice may foresee in implementing the measure, and how that measure may be applied to payment programs. Measures approved by the CMS for implementation in a payment program will most likely undergo at least 3 public comment periods. Measures are often tested and then finalized before submission to the CMS for approval in payment programs or for NQF endorsement.

For practices seeking measures to fit their practice, several publicly available resources describe measures and, in many instances, display complete measure specifications. Quality Payment Program (QPP) measures available for reporting and individual Qualified Clinical Data Registry (QCDR) measures are both required to be publicly available. On other Web sites, such as the Agency for Healthcare Research and Quality Measures Clearinghouse and the NQF Quality Positioning System, practices will find only summaries of measures. The CMS also maintains a Quality Measure warehouse that lists thousands of available quality measures in summary format. For complete measure specifications, practices are encouraged to contact the measure owner or steward listed on each of these Web sites. The practice will be able to identify measures rather quickly through measure searches based on patient condition, care setting, data source, and level of analysis (between clinicians, facilities, and groups). Although benchmarked data may not be publicly available, the practice should contact the listed measure steward to see whether the measure has such benchmarks. In many instances, it would benefit a practice to build a local measure off of a measure found on these Web sites. By doing so, the practice can establish itself in national measurement activities that extend well beyond the walls of their local practice.

Practices contributing data as part of hospital or facility quality initiatives should ask administrators to review the measure logic and algorithms. With many facility-based quality measures, as well as cost and efficiency measures, proper attribution of a patient outcome is obscured or not transparent to the individual practice, let alone the clinician. Because measures used in the Hospital Inpatient Quality Reporting Program, the Hospital Outpatient Quality Reporting Program, the Ambulatory Surgical Center Quality Reporting Program, and many of the other 2 dozen CMS quality programs do not necessarily measure individual practices or clinician actions, it is important that practices learn if and how hospitals and facilities are reporting facility-based quality measures to payers. Ideally, practices and individuals should contact the measure developer and steward on any questions they may have about the measure, including how to collect data and appropriately assess measure performance.

QUALIFIED REGISTRIES AND QUALIFIED CLINICAL DATA REGISTRIES

For purposes of the MIPS, registries must apply with the CMS to accept data as a qualified registry (QR) and/or a QCDR. A QR is an entity that collects clinical data from an individual MIPS-eligible clinician, group, or virtual group and submits it to the CMS on their behalf. For the MIPS Quality Component, clinicians work directly with their chosen QR to submit data on the measures or specialty set of measures they have selected. A QR is limited to reporting MIPS measures.[9] A QCDR is also an entity approved by the CMS that collects clinician's clinical data for submission to the CMS but is different from a QR only in the MIPS Quality Component because QCDR participants may report MIPS and/or QCDR measures (**Table 1**).[10] MIPS quality

Table 1 General 2018 Centers for Medicare & Medicaid Services Qualified Clinical Data Registry and qualified registry self-nomination requirements		
Required Self-Nomination Information	QCDR	QR
Organization name	X	X
New or existing QCDR	X	X
QCDR measure specifications	X	—
Supported MIPS quality measures	X	X
MIPS performance categories	X	X
Performance period	X	X
Vendor type	X	X
How data is captured	X	X
How TINs and National Provider Identifier (NPI) will be verified	X	X
How performance rates for quality measures will be calculated (source of clinician's data)	X	X
Randomized audit process	X	X
Whether validation results will be provided by May 31st after performance period	X	X
Available performance data	X	X
Risk adjustment method for QCDR Measures	X	—

Abbreviation: TIN, tax identification number.

measures are those quality measures that are published in the MIPS regulations and include an anesthesia specialty measure set. QCDR measures are often created by specialty societies or regional quality collaboratives and are approved annually by the CMS. According to current regulations, a QCDR may submit up to 30 QCDR measures for CMS review and approval.[10] To become a CMS-approved QR or QCDR, the organization must undergo rigorous a self-nomination processes each year. This process includes sending all required information through the CMS Web-based tool by the self-nomination deadline.

Because a QR is limited to reporting MIPS measures, once the self-nomination form, measures and data validation plan are approved, a qualified posting is made for the QR on the QPP Web site. The QCDR self-nomination process is similar to the QR except for the additional review of proposed QCDR measures. After the QCDR's self-nomination form and validation plan is approved, the proposed QCDR measures are reviewed by the CMS and are either approved, provisionally approved, or rejected.

REGISTRY DATA CAPTURE AND SUBMISSION

There are many ways for data to make its way into a clinical data registry. Early registries depended on trained data abstractors who extracted the desired data from the medical records, entered the data into certified software or case report forms, and uploaded the data to the registry via a secure Web portal. Although some mature registries such as the STS continue this approach, it is time-consuming and often not a practical option for specialties that cannot depend on the hospital to bear the data abstractor's salary and pay the registry fees. This has required anesthesia and other specialties to develop alternative registry approaches.

In October 2008, the ASA established the Anesthesia Quality Institute (AQI), which developed the National Anesthesia Clinical Outcomes Registry (NACOR), the largest anesthesia registry in the country (https://www.aqihq.org/about-us.aspx). NACOR provides several levels of registry services intended for all anesthesia providers in all practice settings. The NACOR basic service provides interactive analytical reports, the ability to analyze data across various dimensions, and peer-to-peer benchmarks (**Fig. 3**). Outcomes and adverse events, outside of CMS measures, may also be reported.

In addition, physician anesthesiologists and other qualified anesthesia providers in their practices have been using the registry to satisfy federal quality reporting programs. Beginning in 2015, AQI NACOR was an approved QCDR and assisted practices in submitting data for PQRS reporting. When that program ended in 2016, AQI NACOR was an approved QR and QCDR, and submitted data on behalf of individual eligible clinicians and their practices as part of MIPS. In the future, clinical data registries such as AQI NACOR will play a more active and visible role as quality and cost data are increasingly used by the CMS, payers, and other healthcare stakeholders to develop and support participation in APMs.

ANESTHESIA REGISTRY REPORTING CHALLENGES

When it comes to contributing data to a registry, the anesthesia profession faces many unique challenges. First, the proportion of nonoperating room anesthesia care in the United States has increased from 28.3% in 2010 to 35.9% in 2014.[11] The expansion of anesthesia beyond the inpatient hospital operating room means data sources reside in many locations within a hospital, such as invasive radiology, computed tomography and MRI imaging, gastrointestinal endoscopy, electrophysiology, and obstetrics. In addition, anesthesia services are performed in outpatient settings, such

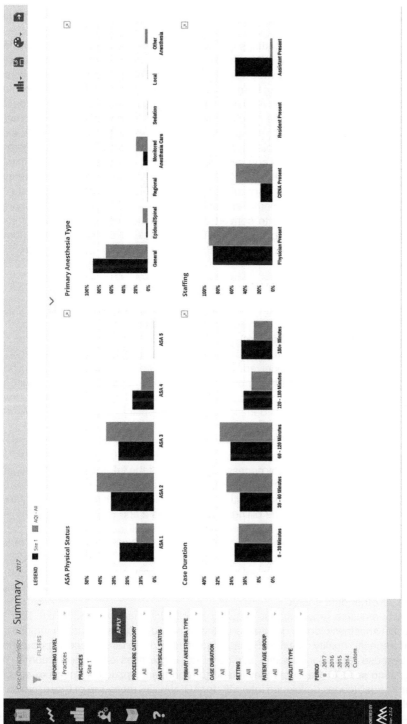

Fig. 3. AQI NACOR sample dashboard report. (*Courtesy of AQI, Schaumburg, IL; and ArborMetrix, Inc, Ann Arbor, MI.*)

as ambulatory surgery centers, office-based surgery centers, and clinics. Finally, making sure that billing data link to electronic anesthesia data and quality data that a practice produces on a patient compounds the challenges in registry reporting.

Just as anesthesia service settings vary widely, so does practice size and business model, both of which affect a practice's ability to successfully participate in a registry. This diversity has resulted in a wide spectrum in the ability of a practice to capture and submit data to a registry, ranging from sophisticated processes at the most technologically advanced academic centers to practices with paper anesthesiology records and charts. It is not unusual for large practices to work with dedicated internal information technology (IT) resources that manage the entire data extraction process from electronic health records (EHRs), billing software, Anesthesia Information Management System (AIMS), and other data sources. However, most practices contract with vendors who provide a range of electronic services, including billing, EHR software integration, and electronic data capture processes through mobile applications for smartphones or tablets. On the other end of the spectrum are the pen-and-paper practices that must use a process to convert their information into an electronic format before it can be submitted to a registry. Data conversion options include manual data entry into a spreadsheet or Web portal, or hiring a vendor to scan paper records.

NATIONAL ANESTHESIA CLINICAL OUTCOMES REGISTRY DATA SOURCES

The billing record is a critical source of information and serves as the backbone of documenting a case. Billing records provide a substantial amount of information that include basic demographic information such as name, date of birth and date of service, as well as insurance status; a patient's diagnosis; and the procedures, services, and supplies a patient has received. Billing records provide the NACOR with codes describing a procedure, generally known as CPT Codes and Healthcare Common Procedure Coding System codes. The claim identifies the clinician providing the service based on the National Provider Identifier, as well as the place of service code. Much of this information is often used to form the denominator or, rather, patient population, for many measures. In other cases, a claim may include different modifiers such as a -1P or -8P that are used to calculate certain exceptions to measure numerators.

However, claims data do not necessarily include all the information that a registry needs for reporting a quality measure. For instance, if a practice is also participating in MIPS quality reporting, several additional data elements, such as the MIPS measure number, are not supplied by the billing record. **Tables 2** and **3** describe the 2017 AQI NACOR Requirements for a minimum data set, as well as additional information needed to report quality measures as part of the MIPS Quality Component. **Table 2** describes the minimum data fields that a practice is required to submit for AQI NACOR to process a measure. Several elements in the table may be taken from claims data but other required data may come from the anesthesia record, a quality capture application, or other data source.

Quality measure reporting also requires specific information to designate that the physician anesthesiologist, qualified anesthesia provider, or their practice intended to report a specific quality measure. Because quality measures target specific populations and because regulations require additional data, practices often must submit data designating specific measures they intend to report, any applicable measure-specific registry codes (codes developed internally for AQI NACOR measures or those measures developed by other registries and measure stewards), and applicable modifiers.

The additional information necessary for processing MIPS quality measures or submission of outcome information is obtained from sources that the NACOR categorizes

Table 2
2017 Anesthesia Quality Institute National Anesthesia Clinical Outcomes Registry minimum data field requirements

Data Elements	Example
Unique anesthesia episode of care identification (ID) number	Alphanumeric value (eg, AM0000123; 1234567; ABC123; 789XYZ123)
Provider TIN	9-character numeric value with preceding zeros (eg, 0234567891; 123456789)
Provider NPI	10-character numeric value, must be a valid NPI the meeting CMS requirements at https://www.cms. gov/Regulations-and-Guidance/Administrative-Simplification/NationalProvidentStand/Downloads/ NPIcheckdigit.pdf
Provider credentials	Advanced Practice Nurse, Anesthesiologist, Certified Anesthesiologist Assistant, Certified Registered Nurse Anesthetist, Fellow (Anesthesiology), Surgeon, Physician Assistant, Registered Nurse, Resident (Anesthesia), Student Registered Nurse Anesthetist, Dentist or Oral Surgeon, Podiatrist
Facility ID (ID created by the practice) Must be the same as the ID provided in the roster (see exhibit a of the participation agreement)	Alphanumeric value (eg, F123, Hospital 1, ASC14)
Date of service	Valid date value in the format YYYY-MM-DD (note, date part of the anesthesia start time)
Anesthesia start time	Date and time when the anesthesia team assumes continuous care of the patient and begins preparing the patient for anesthesia services in the operating room or an equivalent area Combination of the date of service plus anesthesia start time; the ISO 8601 standard for any date and time value is used (YYYY-MM-DDThh:mm:ss [.mmm]->2016-05-01T07:30:00.000)
Anesthesia end time	Date and time when the anesthesiologist turns over care of the patient to a postanesthesia care team (either PACU or ICU). This time ends when the anesthesia team is no longer furnishing anesthesia services to the patient (ie, when the patient may be placed safely under postoperative care and when the anesthesia team has completed transfer of patient care) Combination of the date of service plus anesthesia end time; the ISO 8601 standard for any date and time value is used (YYYY-MM-DDThh:mm:ss [.mmm]->2016-05-01T07:30:00.000)
Patient sex	Male, female, missing, unknown
Patient age, patient date of birth (1 or both)	Patient age: a positive integer between 0 and 130, Patient aged 1 y or less may report as decimal to the 10-thousandths place (eg, a patient aged 5-days old should be reported as 0.0137; 5/365 = 0.0137) Patient date of birth: the month, day, and year on which the patient was born; reported as YYYY-MM-DD

(continued on next page)

Table 2 (continued)	
Data Elements	**Example**
Anesthesia type	Neuraxial, general anesthesia, monitored anesthesia care, peripheral nerve block, no anesthesia provided, unknown
ASA physical status (with E designator when appropriate)	I, IE, II, IIE, III, IIIE, IV, IVE, V, VE, VI
ASA CPT code with modifiers as appropriate	The CPT code set describes medical, surgical, and diagnostic services, and is designed to communicate uniform information about medical services and procedures among physicians, coders, patients, accreditation organizations, and payers for administrative, financial, and analytical purposes 00100–01999; 99100–99150
Surgical CPT codes with modifiers as appropriate	The CPT code set describes medical, surgical, and diagnostic services, and is designed to communicate uniform information about medical services and procedures among physicians, coders, patients, accreditation organizations, and payers for administrative, financial, and analytical purposes 10000–79999; 0000T-9999T
Procedure status	Emergency, urgent, elective, unknown
Payment method	Charity, commercial, government: Medicaid Government: Medicare Fee for Service–Part A Government: Medicare Fee for Service–Part B Government: Medicare Fee for Service–Part C Government: military or veterans Government: other, other, self-pay, unknown, Worker's Compensation

Abbreviations: E, emergent; ICU, intensive care unit; ISO, international organization for standardization; PACU, postanesthesia care unit.

as quality vendors (**Table 3**). These vendors often provide information for the measure numerator indicating whether the measure performance is met. This information may be recorded in paper quality capture forms, pulled from an EHR or AIMS, or captured in specially designed applications using tablets, smartphones, or computers. Information for patient-reported outcomes or patient-satisfaction measures resides outside of the clinical record and are often captured and submitted to NACOR by third-party vendors.

Table 3 Anesthesia Quality Institute National Anesthesia Clinical Outcomes Registry data elements for 2017 Merit-Based Incentive Payment System quality components	
Data Elements	**Examples[a]**
MIPS or QCDR measure number	MIPS 426
Reported value (CPT II code, Healthcare Common Procedure Coding System code, QCDR measure code)	G9656, 10A44
Appropriate code modifiers	1P, 8P, GQ, GT
CMS place of service codes	Numeric value from 01-99

[a] Examples are not inclusive of all applicable data elements.

MERGING DATA FILES

One of the most difficult yet critical steps in successfully submitting data to an anesthesia registry is the process of merging the billing data with the remaining data sources. Depending on whether a practice is reporting outcome data or quality measures for MIPS, data often originate from 2 or 3 different sources. To merge or link these files together, the records from each source must contain a unique anesthesia episode of care identification (ID) number. Ensuring the use of the unique anesthesia episode of care ID across multiple vendors has been an arduous undertaking for many practices because it requires a communication and coordination among the practice and its independent vendors.

Regardless of the collection method or number of data sources, all the data files must be properly merged and formatted before electronic submission to NACOR. In July 2017, AQI introduced a new NACOR data submission portal through which a third-party vendor checks and validates whether the uploaded files adhere to NACOR file requirements (**Fig. 4**). After the data files pass the validation checks, they are then sent to a third-party data warehouse, ArborMetrix, where data are processed and analyzed. Practices log into the NACOR Dashboard provided by ArborMetrix to review the accuracy of the data submitted; confirm the completeness of measures reported (ie, numerator and denominator codes); and, if applicable, whether the data meets quality reporting and performance thresholds. Data warehouse vendors often use a team experienced in healthcare, business, biostatistics, and technology. Data warehouses provide a range of services for registries, including Web-based dashboards, reports and analytical tools, benchmark comparisons, and data formatting and submission to the CMS. Many data warehouses are hosted on Health Insurance Portability and Accountability Act (HIPAA)-compliant cloud-based platforms that adhere to rigorous national standards to ensure operational security as well as participant and patient data and privacy. Significant precautions and contingency planning are used to mitigate the risks associated with data loss and or breaches.

KEYS TO SUCCESSFUL REGISTRY PARTICIPATION

All sizes and types of practices have successfully reported to AQI NACOR. When evaluating AQI NACOR practice performance results for the 2016 PQRS reporting year,

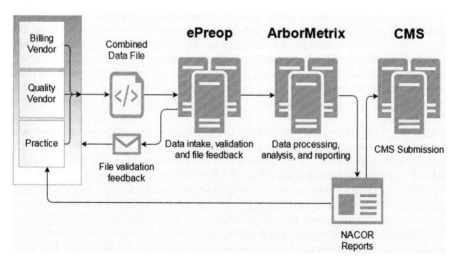

Fig. 4. AQI NACOR 2017 data flow chart. (*Courtesy of* AQI, Schaumburg, IL.)

several factors were identified that affected a practice's success. That year, requirements for successful participation were quite challenging. Physician anesthesiologists and other clinicians required to participate in PQRS had to report 9 quality measures for at least 50% of patients to which the measures applied. This was no small feat for a practice to achieve. The timing of data submission was very important, particularly for small and mid-sized practices and those practices using multiple vendors or a combination of in-house IT staff and a vendor. More often, practices that routinely monitored their NACOR Dashboard for data completeness and compliance with performance thresholds were successful. Practices that either waited to submit data until the deadline or who did not check their NACOR reports throughout the year were less likely to succeed because they did not dedicate sufficient time to identify and correct problems. Vendor performance varied widely and affected which practices were successful. Twenty-five percent of vendors performed very poorly with less than 4% of their client practices successfully submitting data to NACOR. These vendors often struggled with the ability to provide the unique anesthesia episode of care ID necessary for merging files or were unable to submit data in the required format. Forty-one percent of vendors performed very well with greater than 90% of their client practices successfully submitting data to NACOR. Finally, based on AQI observations, practices were more successful when the practice leaders explained the importance of quality reporting, the dollars at risk, and how scores could affect the reputation of an individual or practice.

PRACTICE AND REGISTRY RESPONSIBILITIES

In today's complex reporting world, a turnkey solution to quality reporting would be ideal for many practices and individual physicians. Although many practices may wish that vendors and their medical associations would provide this solution, there are many contingencies that an individual practice may know about that are specific to their practice, for which local knowledge, education, and responsibility are required. There are some key steps that a practice can take to better address their individual reporting needs and instill a greater sense of ownership among their practice participants.

As a basic rule, each practice should and, in many cases, must identify a quality champion, usually an anesthesiologist. However, the role may be delegated to a practice administrator or practice management company. For MIPS reporting, the quality champion is responsible for managing and overseeing the practice's quality reporting activities, including researching and selecting an appropriate reporting mechanism (QR or QCDR), choosing a reporting option (group practice or individual), identifying improvement activities that will be attested to, and identifying the measures that the practice's eligible clinicians will report in the MIPS Quality Component.

After these decisions have been made, the quality champion will need to determine if the practice will use the services of vendors or in-house IT staff to operationalize data collection, formatting, and submission. Even if the quality champion role is delegated to a practice management company, it is very important that someone within the practice gain an understanding of MIPS reporting and performance requirements, coordinate physician and staff training, and meet reporting deadlines. A designated person at the practice level should be responsible for reviewing the NACOR online reports each month, including group and individual performance metrics and quality measure compliance reports. For improvement activities, in particular, the CMS requires a practice to take an active approach to improvement activities and demonstrate that such activities occurred. Each practice is ultimately responsible for ensuring the accuracy of its data and documentation necessary for any audits by the CMS.

A practice champion and practice leadership should also explore how registry reporting can be more than just meeting federal reporting requirements. Registries such as AQI NACOR capture and display data for practices who may not be required to report MIPS but instead wish to see how their performance compares with similar practices. Practices participating in local quality improvement activities should leverage their data collection activities and reporting to AQI NACOR to demonstrate to local hospital administrators the care they provide to individual patients.

For most practices, software vendors play an essential role in the data submission process. Many practices struggle in knowing which questions to ask a vendor, as well as when to ask the questions. In such a competitive environment, vendors should be well-versed in MIPS regulatory requirements and reporting thresholds, and have a clear understanding of the measures it supports. The vendor must be able to meet the NACOR specifications and use the NACOR data definitions. When selecting a vendor, the practice may consider the following:

1. What is the vendor's NACOR reporting success rate?
2. Does the vendor support the measures the practice wishes to report? A billing vendor may need to add fields to capture measure information and commit to yearly measure updates.
3. Does the vendor meet the NACOR formatting requirements?
4. Does the vendor have experience producing a unique anesthesia episode of care ID necessary to merge data from multiple sources?
5. Can the vendor describe examples of collaboration with other vendors or practices related to quality control?

When choosing a registry, anesthesia practices should consider the level of support they will receive related to quality reporting. In addition to supporting MIPS quality and continuous improvement components, AQI provides numerous resources to help practices successfully report data to NACOR. The NACOR User Guide (https://www.aqihq.org/files/2017_NACOR_User_Guide_Final_10.31.17.pdf) is among the most useful resources AQI annually produces. This guide provides an online step-by-step description to submitting data to the NACOR. The NACOR User Guide is supplemented by monthly virtual Webinars during office hours, recorded training materials, weekly NACOR News, including updates, deadline reminders, and answers to frequently asked questions. NACOR participants may submit questions via an online user help desk or may contact their personal NACOR account representatives. Online NACOR reports are always available and assistance with report interpretation is available on request.

QUALITY REPORTING

In the past few decades, the burden of quality reporting on practices has grown as more facility administers and payers demand that practices and individual clinicians be held to a higher standard of patient care. Although this burden has increased, the use of the technology and registries has filled a gap in collecting, reporting, and analyzing practice data. Such data help measure developers and stewards to identify future measures needed as healthcare delivery transitions to a value-based payment system. Quality reporting, whether as part of national payment programs or for local improvement activities, will continue to be a core requirement for practices of all sizes and clinicians from all specialties.

REFERENCES

1. Centers for Medicare & Medicaid Services. Blueprint for the CMS measures management system. vol. 13. Baltimore (MD): Centers for Medicare & Medicaid Services; 2017.
2. The Joint Commission. Specifications manual for National Hospital inpatient quality measures, version 5.1. Oak Brook (IL): The Joint Commission; 2016. p. v–xii.
3. Center for Clinical Standards and Quality Centers for Medicare & Medicaid Services. CMS quality measure development plan: supporting the transition to the quality payment Program 2017 Annual Report. 2017. p. 1.
4. Centers for Medicare & Medicaid Services. 2015 reporting experience including trends (2007-2015): physician quality reporting system. Baltimore (MD): Centers for Medicare & Medicaid Services; 2017. p. 4. Appendix Table A16.
5. Center for Clinical Standards and Quality Centers for Medicare & Medicaid Services. CMS quality measure development plan: supporting the transition to the quality payment program 2017 Annual Report. Current activities of the Care Quality Measures Collaborative can be accessed on the CMS Web site. 2017. p. 14. Available at: https://www.cms.gov/Medicare/Quality-Initiatives-Patient-Assessment-Instruments/QualityMeasures/Core-Measures.html. Accessed March 11, 2018.
6. National Quality Forum. NQF's history. Available at: https://www.qualityforum.org/about_nqf/history/. Accessed November 13, 2017.
7. National Quality Forum. Funding. Available at: https://www.qualityforum.org/About_NQF/Funding.aspx. Accessed November 13, 2017.
8. National Quality Forum. NQF: consensus development process. Available at: https://www.qualityforum.org/Measuring_Performance/Consensus_Development_Process.aspx. Accessed October 19, 2017.
9. Centers for Medicare & Medicaid Services. 2018 Merit-based Incentive Payment System (MIPS) Qualified Registry Self-Nomination Fact Sheet. Baltimore (MD): Centers for Medicare & Medicaid Services; 2017. Available at: https://www.cms.gov/Medicare/Quality-Initiatives-Patient-Assessment-Instruments/Value-Based-Programs/MACRA-MIPS-and-APMs/2018-Registry-fact-sheet-.pdf. Accessed November 12, 2017.
10. Centers for Medicare & Medicaid Services. 2018 Merit-based Incentive Payment System (MIPS) Qualified Clinical Data Registry (QCDR) Self-Nomination Fact Sheet. Baltimore (MD): Centers for Medicare & Medicaid Services; 2017. Available at: https://www.cms.gov/Medicare/Quality-Initiatives-Patient-Assessment-Instruments/Value-Based-Programs/MACRA-MIPS-and-APMs/2018-QCDR-fact-sheet-.pdf. Accessed November 12, 2017.
11. Nagrebetsky A, Gabriel RA, Dutton RP, et al. Growth of nonoperating room anesthesia care in the United States: a contemporary trends analysis. Anesth Analg 2017;124(4):1261–7.

Quality and the Health System

Becoming a High Reliability Organization

Monaliza Gaw, MPA, MSN, CPHQ, NEA-BC, RN[a],
Frank Rosinia, MD, MHCM[a,b,*], Thomas Diller, MD, MMM[c,1]

KEYWORDS

- Safety • Reliability • Culture • Microsystems • HRO • High reliability organizations
- Patient safety culture

KEY POINTS

- Despite substantial improvement efforts, health care quality and patient safety lag behind the expected level of performance; medical errors are the third leading cause of death in the United States.
- Improvements in quality and patient safety require the transition to the concepts of high reliability organizing used in many other complex industries.
- High reliability organizing is focused on leadership commitment, dedication to a culture of safety, and the use of advanced performance improvement methods.
- Leaders must engage clinical microsystems to successfully build and implement the concepts of high reliability organizing.

INTRODUCTION

Each day, hundreds of thousands of physicians, nurses, therapists, and other health care providers come to work with the intention of providing excellent care to the patients they serve. Before the 1990s, it was assumed that health care was a safe and high-quality endeavor. Errors that were occasionally recognized were assumed to be due to the actions of specific providers who carelessly made mistakes. Thus,

Disclosure Statement: No disclosures to report.
[a] JPS Heath Network, 1500 South Main Street, Fort Worth, TX 76104, USA; [b] Department of Health Behavior and Health Systems, School of Public Health, University of North Texas Health Science Center, 3500 Camp Bowie Boulevard, EAD 402, Fort Worth, TX 76107, USA; [c] Department of Health Behavior and Health Systems, School of Public Health, University of North Texas Health Science Center, Institute for Patient Safety, 3500 Camp Bowie Boulevard, EAD 402, Fort Worth, TX 76107, USA
[1] Senior author.
* Corresponding author. 3604 Dorothy Lane, Fort Worth, TX 76107.
E-mail address: frankrosinia@me.com

Anesthesiology Clin 36 (2018) 217–226
https://doi.org/10.1016/j.anclin.2018.01.010
1932-2275/18/© 2018 Elsevier Inc. All rights reserved.

most of the quality and patient safety efforts centered on mortality and morbidity reviews and peer review to identify and remediate those health care providers that were not high quality. With the publication of the Institute of Medicine's reports, "To Err is Human" in 1999 and "Crossing the Quality Chasm" in 2001, the perspective that all mistakes were made by poor training, intention, or negligence began to change.[1,2] Now, nearly 2 decades into intense quality and patient safety improvement work, we collectively have a much better understanding of the true impact and causation for suboptimal quality and medical error.

Over the past 2 decades, there have been many pivotal revelations. For example, Dr. Elizabeth McGlynn and her associates published the landmark article, "The Quality of Health Care Delivered to Adults in the United States" in 2003 that demonstrated only 55% compliance with 439 process indicators that were considered to be evidence based.[3] Numerous papers originated from Fisher and Wennberg[4–6] working on the Dartmouth Atlas that demonstrated pervasive unwarranted variation in the delivery of medical care in various geographies. These variations were counter to the goal to provide care that was evidence based and rather due to organizational and economic factors unrelated to patient need. Further, these variations were associated with substantial regional variations in cost. However, spending more on health care failed to produce improvements in quality, access to care, and or patient satisfaction. In 2010 and 2011, 3 pivotal and systematic papers were published that together demonstrated adverse event rates in hospitalized patients ranging between 18% and 33%, with up to 1.5% of those patients suffering a lethal outcome.[7–9] This work culminated in the landmark article published in 2016 by Makary and Daniel[10] that estimated medical error in hospitalized patients causes approximately 251,000 deaths per year, making it the third leading cause of death in the United States behind only heart disease and cancer.

We currently live and work within a health care system that produces some of the most amazing outcomes possible. There have been incredible advances in heart disease, cancer, trauma, and many other services. The US delivery system has the ability to perform miracles for countless patients each year. Yet, sadly, we continue to fail to provide evidence-based and safe care routinely. Much has been written about both our superb accomplishments and the causes of our failures. In 2010, Mark Chassin and Jerod Loeb[11] at The Joint Commission called for radical change, strongly arguing the health care delivery system must transition from peer review and project-based improvement efforts to embrace the concepts of high reliability organizing that is so prevalent and effective in many other high-risk industries.

HIGH RELIABILITY ORGANIZATIONS

Reliability is the probability that a system will yield a specified result. Thus, high reliability organizations are those organizations that are involved in a complex, high-risk environment that deliver exceptional safety and consistency every day. Chassin and Loeb outlined a framework for high reliability based on the successes of other industries such as the military, commercial aviation, and nuclear power. Becoming an high reliability organization cannot be approached as a project with a checklist of things to accomplish that ultimately results in the achievement of high reliability status. Rather, the work is a constant journey toward excellence. The more appropriate definition of an high reliability organization, therefore, is high reliability organizing — the constant organization of work and infrastructure that leads to highly reliable outcomes.

Chassin and Loeb's framework focused on leadership, safety culture, and robust performance improvement methods. Within this context, leadership refers to a very conscious effort by both senior and front-line leaders, in both words and actions, to center the organization's mission, vision, and values on principles that will lead to high reliability. The most important thing health care organizations do every day is to deliver high-quality, safe care to those patients who have entrusted us with their very lives. Thus, both administrative and clinical leaders have the ethical imperative to act consistently with our mission and values in every decision we make. Second, health care organizations must radically change their safety culture to one in which all team members constantly act with the same ethical imperative to deliver high-quality and safe care. Finally, they argued that the performance improvement methods often used are wholly inadequate for the complexity of the operations and clinical problems we are asked to address on a daily basis. Evidence suggests that we must understand these complexities to craft solutions capable of solving problems and creating efficient, highly reliable work processes. Functionally, this means moving away from copying solutions from other organizations and the use of less robust performance improvement methods such as plan–do–check–act toward the use of robust methods such as lean, 6 sigma, and change management.

Health care organizations are just now beginning to embrace quality and safety science that is well-established in other industries. Critical for success is fully embracing the work of James Reason and his lifelong learning regarding error causation.[12,13] Organizations produce their work through a myriad of processes, each of which is designed to achieve a specific outcome. In Reason's study of error causation, he noted that errors occur owing to either the failure of systems and processes and/or the failure of humans. Processes typically have built-in defense barriers to prevent system error and to prevent and mitigate inevitable human error. These defense barriers also have inherent weaknesses. Thus, when adverse events occur, typically, it is not due to a bad person, but rather due to both system and human errors that accumulate and overcome the defense barriers. Adverse events then have multiple root causes, each of which must be understood and specifically corrected. A systematic study of health care adverse events using Reasons approach has been published, "HFACS Applied to Health Care," and recently, the National Patient Safety Foundation published an excellent summary approach to adverse event investigation, "RCA^2 Improving Root Cause Analyses ad Actions to Prevent Harm."[14,15]

Finally, no discussion of high reliability is complete without a review of Weick and Sutcliffe's landmark study, "Managing the Unexpected: Resilient Performance in an Age of Uncertainty."[16] In this book, they studied numerous organizations and outlined the concepts of collectivity, collective mindfulness, and collective enactment. Collectivity refers to similar behaviors that everyone in an organization manifests. Collective mindfulness refers to a cultural way of thinking in which people are educated on the systems they work within and are constantly evaluating their environment and the functioning of those systems. Thus, they become aware in real time when errors might be about to occur. Organizations commonly operate under a set of expectations to create orderliness and predictability. Expectations can create blind spots during our work when we fail to recognize unexpected threatening events. These blind spots can grow when we search for evidence to confirm our original bias. Expectations about how work should be conducted means that we are ready for work to happen in that way. We are mentally ready to see work unfold in a certain manner. High reliability organizations are able to counteract these blind spots by developing a greater awareness of discriminatory detail. Collective mindfulness is the antidote for being taken by surprise. It is manifested in organizations when everyone is acutely aware that small failures in processes can lead to disastrous outcomes. Collective enactment refers to a cultural paradigm such that, when people become aware that something might be amiss, they immediately and intentionally change their work to address the issue and correct it.

Weick and Sutcliffe further describe 5 key concepts that are present in high reliability organizing. These include:

- *Sensitivity to operations:* Both management and staff understand their systems and processes, how they are designed to work and what might go wrong. Further, they are constantly aware of how their systems are performing.
- *Reluctance to simplify:* Although systems and processes are made as simple as possible, when failure occurs, high reliability organizations refuse simple explanations for the failure. Instead, they rigorously pursue and understand each failed system.
- *Preoccupation with failure*: High reliability organizations maintain a relentless pursuit of perfection. They are convinced the next error is about to happen and are constantly searching for what might go wrong.
- *Deference to expertise*: Leaders listen and respond to the insights of the front line. Additionally, in an urgent situation or crisis, the person with the greatest expertise for that situation leads, regardless of rank or title.
- *Resilience*: Humans and systems make mistakes and things will go wrong. High reliability organizations are able to quickly identify an adverse event is occurring and makes successful efforts to rapidly contain and mitigate the error. Leaders and staff are trained and well-prepared to know how to respond when system failures occur.

The health care industry is learning the value of high reliability principles that have a proven track record of success in the nuclear power industry, commercial air travel, and military aircraft carriers.[17] Malcolm Gladwell teaches us about the foundational significance of communication for safety in the airline industry in his book, *Outliers: The Story of Success*. The fatal crash of Avianca flight 052 in January of 1990 occurs when Captain Laureano Caviedes was attempting to land his plane en route from Medellin, Columbia, to New York City's Kennedy Airport. Poor weather had caused numerous flight delays up and down the East Coast. While attempting to land flight 052 was asked to circle over Norfolk, Virginia, above Atlantic City, and above Kennedy Airport. When the captain was finally given permission to land, severe wind shear forced the plane to pull up and execute a "go-around" over Long Island, New York. Suddenly an engine failed and then the second engine failed and the plane crashed in a posh estate in the town of Oyster Bay on Long Island. Seventy-three of the 158 passengers aboard died. The cause of the crash was fuel exhaustion. There was nothing mechanically wrong with the plane and the pilots were sober. When the black box was recovered, it was found that the cockpit was filled with long stretches of silence up until the time of the crash. The captain and first officer understood the urgency of their fuel level, but failed to effectively communicate this to air traffic control. How could this happen? The airline industry learned from this and many other fatal crashes that effective and timely communication is a prerequisite for safety. Hierarchy and silence in the cockpit can cause airline crashes. Today every major airline uses crew resource management training to teach junior crewmembers how to communicate clearly and assertively. What can health care learn from the airline industry?

COMMUNICATION AND PATIENT SAFETY

Amy Edmonson has been at the forefront of the discussion in health care studying how psychological safety and communication translate into patient safety.[18–21] In a psychologically safe environment, team members are safe to speak up, admit a mistake, or challenge a process. Individuals in a psychologically safe health care organization believe that they will not be punished or disciplined for taking risks to discuss problems and report errors. Employees feel safe to discuss near misses and adverse events so others can learn and improvement can occur. An example that illustrates a psychologically safe culture occurred during the night shift on a postpartum unit. A nurse mistakenly gave a mother stored breast milk from a common refrigerator that was not her own. The nurse quickly realized her mistake, retrieved the mistaken breast milk, and reported the incident to the day shift at morning report. The nurse was praised for bringing the issue forward by her supervisor and a system defect that caused the breast milk event was identified. If this had occurred on a nursing unit with a psychologically unsafe environment, the event would not have been reported and a learning opportunity missed. This type of voluntary incident reporting correlates directly with a culture of patient safety.[22] The better the culture of safety, the greater the volume of voluntary reporting on patient safety events. A psychologically safe environment will facilitate interpersonal risk-taking behavior that promotes innovation and patient safety. Psychological safety creates an environment within the team that encourages communication, supports productive conflict, increases accountability, and promotes innovation. A culture of incivility in the workplace has deleterious effects on the performance of medical teams.[23] Daniel Buccino, the director of the Johns Hopkins Civility Initiative, defines civility as "a sense of respect for one's self and for others. Incivility occurs when rude and disrespectful behaviors become prevalent. Sometimes that means making one's own thoughts, wishes and privileges secondary to others."[24] Rudeness and incivility were found to debilitate the collaborative mechanisms recognized as essential for patient care and safety. These included consequences on diagnostic and intervention parameters, information sharing, helping, and communication (**Fig. 1**). The effectiveness of our communication and leadership in health care has consequences for our patients and the well-being of employees.

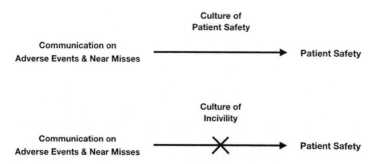

Fig. 1. The influence of culture on communication in an organization.

Leadership has been recognized as an important element for the creation of a psychologically safe climate.[25] Leaders creates the work environment by controlling aspects of interpersonal relationships and communication. Autocratic leaders deter followers from expressing concerns and reporting errors, whereas inclusive leaders encourage a climate for communication.[26] Communication facilitates team learning. In the airline industry, improvements in communication created record improvements in airline safety. Psychological safety acts as a mediator between leadership and team learning. Leader behaviors are key to follower perceptions about the risks associated with speaking up.

Edmondson has described key leadership behaviors for cultivating psychological safety and high-performance teaming and learning[25]:

- *Be accessible and approachable:* Leaders encourage team members to learn together by being accessible and personally involved.
- *Acknowledge the limits of current knowledge:* When leaders admit that they do not know something, their genuine display of humility encourages other team members to follow suit.
- *Be willing to display fallibility:* To create psychological safety, team leaders must demonstrate a tolerance of failure by acknowledging their own fallibility.
- *Invite participation:* When people believe their leaders value their input, they are more engaged and responsive.
- *Highlight failures as learning opportunities:* Instead of punishing people for well-intentioned risks that backfire, leaders encourage team members to embrace error and deal with failure in a productive manner.
- *Use direct language:* Using direct, actionable language instigates the type of straightforward, blunt discussion that enables learning.
- *Set boundaries:* When leaders are as clear as possible about what is acceptable, people feel more psychologically safe then when boundaries are vague or unpredictable.
- *Hold people accountable for transgressions:* When people cross boundaries set in advance and fail to perform up to set standards, leaders must hold them accountable in a fair and consistent way.

Leaders should let employees know they respect employees by routinely acknowledging their expertise and skills. Employees should be rewarded when they speak up and report mistakes. Autocratic leaders will make employees reluctant to share ideas or mistakes. These recommendations hold for all leaders in health care organizations, especially middle managers, who are close to frontline employees directly involved in patient care. Leaders in health care organizations have the ability to establish organizational culture. Signals sent by those in power are key to shaping the willingness of others to speak about events and issues that can improve care and create a culture of patient safety.

Cultivating psychological safety and engaging frontline employees directly involved in patient care creates an environment that fosters an increased awareness of safety or events that can impact safety. To this end, linking high reliability organization principles with a microsystem perspective is integral in the improvement journey. An organization that practices collective mindfulness consistently engages in a "radical presentness" and a mindset that something can go wrong.[27] Nelson and associates posit a theoretic framework that uses microsystems in health care.

A clinical microsystem is defined as a small group of people who work together on a regular basis to provide care to discrete subpopulations of patients. It has clinical and business aims, linked processes, and a shared information environment, and it produces performance outcomes. Microsystems evolve over time and are often embedded in larger organizations.[27]

Although the link between high reliability organization principles and the microsystem involves other factors, the concept of high reliability organizations suggests that team and individual performance depends on the development of organizational norms. Through the extensive experience of Nelson and colleagues working with multiple microsystems, they offer key safety principles that can be used for embedding patient safety concepts with clinical microsystems[28]:

Principle 1 – Errors are human nature and will happen because humans are not infallible.
Principle 2 – The microsystem is the unit of analysis and training.
Principle 3 – Design systems to identify, prevent, absorb, and mitigate errors.
Principle 4 – Create a culture of safety.
Principle 5 – Talk with and listen to patients.
Principle 6 – Integrate practices from human factors engineering into microsystem functioning.

These principles support Amy Edmonson's description of leadership behaviors that foster psychological safety.[25] Additionally, an environment that encourages the reporting of near misses and adverse events promotes a culture of safety through the lens of learning.

ANESTHESIOLOGY

Anesthesiology has been on the forefront of quality, safety, and high reliability much longer than most other specialties in health care. Through careful attention to systems and processes and human factor engineering, deaths owing to anesthesia have been reduced to 6 sigma levels of quality and safety.[29] Opportunities for improvement still exist. Recent surveys, for example, show a pervasive practice to reuse syringes and, in some cases, needles, on multiple patients by anesthesia personnel.[30,31] Anesthesiologists work in a complex environment where there is high interdependence and continuous change.[32] The high reliability organization principles adapt particularly well to complex environments like the operating room. Small problems that are easily overlooked can become a big problem that can be of consequence to our patients. Anesthesiologists have key interdependent roles with surgeons, operating room nurses, operating room techs, nurse anesthetists, and colleagues. This complex interdependence is similar to the setting of an aircraft carrier. The work of anesthesiologists is nonroutine and complex. Adaption of the high reliability organization paradigm is necessary and beneficial to our patients when they are in a vulnerable state. Christianson and colleagues[33] outline how the principles of a high reliability organization can be applied to an intensive care unit (**Table 1**). It is a logical evolution to adopt these concepts to our work as anesthesiologists in the operating room. The safety of our patients would benefit.

By embracing the principles of high reliability, safety science, and robust performance improvement methods to further optimize culture, we can make health care safer and of higher quality for all patients we serve.

Table 1
Principles of high reliability organizing applied to the ICU and OR

Principle	Applications in the ICU and OR
Preoccupation with failure	Postcode and postoperative debriefings. Likely mechanisms of a patient's decomposition at shift change or relief in the OR. Engage in regular performance benchmarking. Establish a psychologically safe culture to encourage reporting of near misses and failures. Use detailed analysis of incidents and errors for potential improvements in processes.
Reluctance to simplify	Be aware of cognitive bias in diagnosis and clinical care. Use multidisciplinary analyses as a basis for decision making. Use team-based analysis for care based decision making. Resist the tendency to assign only 1 cause to incidents and errors.
Sensitivity to operations	Maintain awareness of the patient's overall condition rather than a focus on one problem or organ system. Use tools that facilitate information sharing between team members. Monitor unit, OR, and hospital-based conditions such as bed availability, drug shortages, and personnel absences.
Resilience	Emphasize the importance of working together in teams. Encourage team members to accommodate changes in patient acuity and hospital resources. Include training around how to manage unexpected events in the ICU and OR.
Deference to expertise	Foster knowledge of team members' particular strengths and weaknesses. Use clinical pathways that leverage all levels of expertise (nurse-driven sedation, respiratory therapist-led weaning protocols). Institute multidisciplinary rounds and preoperative briefs which that include all team members and families.

Abbreviations: ICU, intensive care unit; OR, operating room.
Adapted from Christianson MK, Sutcliffe KM, Miller MA, et al. Becoming a high reliability organization. Crit Care 2011;15(6):314; with permission.

REFERENCES

1. Kohn L, Corrigan J, Donaldson M, editors. To err is human: building a safer health system. Washington, DC: National Academy Press; 1999.
2. Institute of Medicine. Crossing the quality chasm a new health system for the 21st century. Washington, DC: National Academy Press; 2001.
3. McGlynn EA, Asch SM, Adams J, et al. The quality of health care delivered to adults in the United States. N Engl J Med 2003;348:2635–45.
4. Fisher ES, Wennberg DE, Stukel TA, et al. The Implications of regional variations in Medicare spending. Part 1: the content, quality, and accessibility of care. Ann Intern Med 2003;138(4):273–87.
5. Fisher ES, Wennberg DE, Stukel TA, et al. The implications of regional variations in Medicare spending. Part 2: health outcomes and satisfaction with care. Ann Intern Med 2003;138(4):288–98.
6. Fisher E, Goodman D, Skinner J, et al. Health care spending, quality, and outcomes: more isn't always better. The Dartmouth Institute for Health Policy & Clinical Practice; 2009. Available at: http://www.dartmouthatlas.org/downloads/reports/Spending_Brief_022709.pdf. Accessed October 5, 2017.

7. Landrigan CP, Parry GJ, Bones CB, et al. Temporal trends in rates of patient harm resulting from medical care. N Engl J Med 2010;363:2124–34.
8. Levinson DR. Adverse events in hospitals: national incidence among Medicare beneficiaries. Department of Health and Human Services: Office of Inspector General; 2010. Available at: https://oig.hhs.gov/oei/reports/oei-06-09-00090.pdf. Accessed October 5, 2017.
9. Classen DC, Resar R, Griffin F, et al. 'Global Trigger Tool' shows that adverse events in hospitals may be ten times greater than previously measured. Health Aff 2011;30(4):581–9.
10. Makary MA, Daniel M. Medial error—the third leading cause of death in the US. BMJ 2016;353:i2139.
11. Chassin MR, Loeb JM. The ongoing quality improvement journey: next stop, high reliability. Health Aff 2011;30(4):559–68.
12. Reason J. Human error. Cambridge (United Kingdom): Cambridge University Press; 1990.
13. Reason J. Managing the risks of organizational accidents. Burlington (VT): Ashgate Publishing; 1997.
14. Diller T, Helmrich G, Dunning S, et al. The Human Factors Analysis Classification System (HFACS) applied to health care. Am J Med Qual 2013;29(3):181–90.
15. National Patient Safety Foundation. RCA^2 improving root cause analyses and actions to prevent harm. 2016. Available at: http://c.ymcdn.com/sites/www.npsf.org/resource/resmgr/PDF/RCA2_v2 online-pub_010816.pdf. Accessed October 5, 2017.
16. Weick KE, Sutcliffe KM. Managing the unexpected: resilient performance in an age of uncertainty. San Francisco (CA): Wiley & Sons; 2007.
17. Gladwell M. Outliers the story of success. New York: Little, Brown and Company; 2008.
18. Edmondson A. Learning from mistakes is easier said than done: group and organizational influences on the detection and correction of human error. J Appl Behav Sci 1996;32(1):5–28.
19. Edmondson AC. Psychological safety and learning behavior in work teams. Adm Sci Q 1999;44(2):350–83.
20. Edmondson AC. Speaking up in the operating room: how team leaders promote learning in interdisciplinary action teams. J Manag Stud 2003;40(6):1419–52.
21. Edmondson AC, Lei Z. Psychological safety: the history, renaissance, and future of an interpersonal construct. Annu Rev Organ Psychol Organ Behav 2014;1(1):23–43.
22. Weingart SN, Farbstein K, Davis RB, et al. Using a multihospital survey to examine the safety culture. Jt Comm J Qual Saf 2004;30(3):125–32.
23. Riskin A, Erez A, Foulk T, et al. Rudeness and medical team performance. Pediatrics 2017;139(2):1–11.
24. Minkove J. Q & A with Daniel Buccino minding our manners. Dome; 2017. p. 7.
25. Edmondson AC. Teaming how organizations learn, innovate, and compete in the knowledge economy. San Francisco (CA): John Wiley & Sons; 2012.
26. Derickson R, Fishman J, Osatuke K, et al. Psychological safety and error reporting within veterans health administration hospitals. J Patient Saf 2014;11(1):60–6.
27. Nelson E, Batalden P, Godfrey M. Quality by design: a clinical microsystems approach. San Francisco (CA): Wiley & Sons; 2007.
28. Trustees of Dartmouth College, Godfrey M, Nelson E, Batalden P. The clinical microsystem action guide. 2004. Available at: http://clinicalmicrosystem.org/wp-content/uploads/2014/07/CMAG040104.pdf. Accessed October 7, 2017.

29. Li G, Warner M, Lang BH, et al. Epidemiology of anesthesia-related mortality in the United States, 1999-2005. Anesthesiology 2009;110(4):759–65.
30. Ford K. Survey of syringe and needle safety among student registered nurse anesthetists: are we making any progress? AANA J 2013;81(1):37–42. Available at: http://web.a.ebscohost.com/ehost/pdfviewer/pdfviewer?vid=2&sid=5277866e-e7a6-49a7-afd7-ae3b66465dd1%40sessionmgr4008.
31. Kossover-Smith RA, Coutts K, Hatfield KM, et al. One needle, one syringe, only one time? A survey of physician and nurse knowledge, attitudes, and practices around injection safety. Am J Infect Control 2017;45:1018–23.
32. Sutcliff K. High reliability organizations (HROs). Best Pract Res Clin Anesthesiol 2011;25:133–44.
33. Christianson MA, Sutcliff K, Miller M, et al. Becoming a high reliability organization. Crit Care 2011;15:314.

Section III: Anesthesiology's Value Proposition

Value Proposition and Anesthesiology

Joseph W. Szokol, MD, JD, MBA[a,b,*], Keith J. Chamberlin, MD, MBA[c]

KEYWORDS

- Value proposition • HCAHPS • Value-based purchasing
- Perioperative surgical home • Anesthesia management companies
- Patient satisfaction

KEY POINTS

- The rapidly evolving anesthesia landscape will place greater pressures than ever on anesthesia practices to deliver high quality care at the lowest possible cost.
- Anesthesia groups must deliver value to their organization by being good corporate citizens and providing value by service, availability, and customer satisfaction.
- It is vital that anesthesia practices institute the Perioperative Surgical Home (PSH), or a portion thereof, to improve value, and provide better results at a lower cost.
- It is important for each practice to develop a strategic plan by using an SWOT (Strengths, Weaknesses, Opportunities, and Threats) analysis to better know how their group stacks up in a hypercompetitive environment.
- There has been a cataclysmic shift in the anesthesia market with large anesthesia management companies comprising some 20% of the anesthesia market and it is important to understand the reasons this has occurred.

WHY DOES AN ANESTHESIA GROUP NEED A VALUE PROPOSITION?

We live in the ever-changing and economically adverse world of Request for Proposal for Anesthesia Services (RFPs), decreasing stipends, and increasing demands. Clinical excellence is expected, and it is a given that your anesthesia group meets or exceeds all quality benchmarks. A group needs to go beyond just delivering quality clinical services. It must additionally serve as good corporate citizens, providing value

Disclosure Statement: J.W. Szokol has no disclosures. K.J. Chamberlin is a member of the Principal Chamberlin Health Care Consulting Group.
[a] Department of Anesthesiology, Critical Care and Pain Medicine, NorthShore University HealthSystem, 2650 Ridge Avenue, Room 3106, Evanston, IL 60201, USA; [b] Pritzker School of Medicine, University of Chicago, 5841 South Maryland Avenue, MC 4028, Chicago, IL 60637, USA; [c] Chamberlin Health Care Consulting Group, 540 San Pedro Cove, San Rafael, CA 94901, USA
* Corresponding author. Department of Anesthesiology, Critical Care and Pain Medicine, North-Shore University HealthSystem, Evanston Hospital, 2650 Ridge Avenue, Room 3106, Evanston, IL 60201.
E-mail address: szokolmd@gmail.com

in a myriad of ways, such as service, availability, customer (patients, surgeons, administrators) satisfaction, and so forth. We do that, so why doesn't the hospital chief executive officer (CEO) know that? Because we are terrible at effectively communicating our enormous value and many contributions as compared with our cost. That is the Value Proposition.

THE VALUE PROPOSITION

Very likely you have seen the equation in **Fig. 1** over and over again, as medicine moves to "value-based care." It is one of the concepts to help you develop your strategy to compete within your market. We will use several business concepts to create a strong value proposition for your practice.

The term "value proposition" was originally coined in 1988 in a staff paper written by the consulting firm McKinsey.[1] It defined a value proposition as "*a clear, simple statement of the benefits, both tangible and intangible, that the company will provide, along with the approximate price it will charge each customer segment for those benefits*.

That is the official version. The down and dirty version is when you are constructing your value proposition, you need to think like your customer: WIIFM or *"what's in it for me?"* Why on earth should I hire *this* anesthesia group? What motivates me to specifically use you (**Fig. 2**)?

Always remember you are in a competitive market, and do not think for a minute that legal remedies will protect you from being replaced (exclusive contracts). At all times, your group must offer superior perceived benefits at a perceived reasonable cost. A start is with an analysis of your group.

UNDERSTAND YOUR BUSINESS

Developing a successful value proposition comes from understanding your group and market environment. What are your strengths and weaknesses (internal to the group) and what are your threats and opportunities (external to the group)? What resources and capabilities can the group use to develop a competitive advantage? This is what an SWOT analysis is all about (**Fig. 3**): looking at your group's strengths, weaknesses, opportunities, and threats.

Box 1 provides some examples.

Strengths

Value is more than just giving anesthesia. How are you viewed by the surgeons and the hospital? How do you *want* to be viewed? What do you offer as a perceived benefit?

Weaknesses

Be honest with yourself here. The most common reason an RFP is issued is because anesthesia groups cannot control or discipline the bad actors and disruptive physicians within their group.

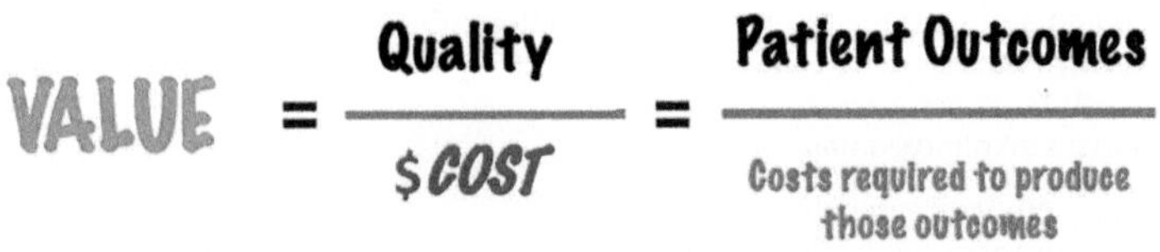

$$\text{VALUE} = \frac{\text{Quality}}{\$COST} = \frac{\text{Patient Outcomes}}{\text{Costs required to produce those outcomes}}$$

Fig. 1. The value proposition.

$$\text{Motivation} = \text{Perceived Benefits} - \text{Perceived Costs}$$

Fig. 2. Motivation.

Opportunities: Leadership, Patient Satisfaction, Perioperative Surgical Home

It becomes paramount that the person leading the group has the requisite leadership skills, emotional intelligence, negotiations, and financial tools available to guide the group forward. The American Society of Anesthesiologists (ASA) has many programs, as do external organizations, such as American College of Healthcare Executives, that can help group leadership obtain the skills and knowledge to lead effectively. Opportunities within the ASA abound to improve one's ability to lead. These opportunities may be obtained through courses such as the ASA Certificate in Business Administration (CBA), ASA-Kellogg School of Management at Northwestern University joint venture on executive physician leadership skills, and the ASA Committee on Practice Management's annual meeting. All of these look at a myriad of issues facing the anesthesiologist. Allowing group leadership to stay in a position for a prolonged period of time, rather than rotating every year or 2, gives that individual more time to develop relationships with hospital administration, nursing, and surgeons. This knowledge and trust become even more critical at times of hospital renegotiation of services contract.

Satisfaction surveys are important tools that help quantify how your group (and individual department members) is looked at by patients, surgeons, and nursing. Literature is emerging that patient satisfaction may very well be tied to quality. Patient experience is a valid dimension of health care quality, as **Table 1** demonstrates. Hospitals with the

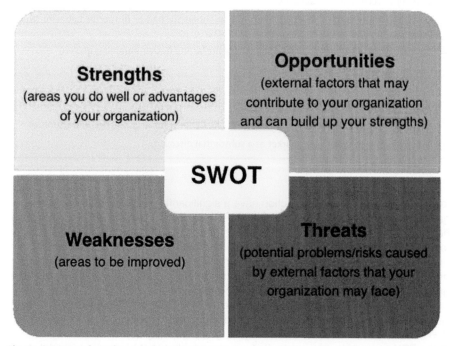

Fig. 3. SWOT analysis. (*From* Kyle B. SWOT analysis—strengths, weaknesses, opportunities, and threats. All about marketing skills. Available at: http://marketing-skills.blogspot.com/2014/09/swot-analysis-strengths-weaknesses.html. Accessed January 30, 2018; with permission.)

Box 1
Examples of SWOT (strengths, weaknesses, opportunities, and threats) analysis

Strengths:

- Physician-anesthesiologists are board certified or board eligible
- Full staffing roster to cover all anesthetizing locations without delays
- Leaders with business acumen or official business credentials
- History of excellent cooperation with regulatory agencies
- Fiscally responsible: looking for ways to decrease hospital costs
  - Streamlined preoperative process
  - All or part of a perioperative surgical home!
  - Acting like a hospital "partner"
- Offer fellowship trained specialty care (ie, pediatrics, cardiac, obstetrics)
- Offer advanced ultrasound-guided peripheral nerve blocks
- CEO never hears complaints about "anesthesia"
- You measure and act on results of an ongoing patient satisfaction survey

Opportunities:

- Filling a missing need in your market (endoscopy, radiology sedation, new technology)
- Sending group leaders to business classes, CBA, MBA, Leadership training, and so forth
- New surgicenters or physician offices that could benefit from formal sedation

Weaknesses:

- Inability to recruit and retain outstanding physician-anesthesiologists and/or CRNAs
- Lack of structure to be able discipline group members for bad or disruptive behavior (this being the number 1 reason groups lose contracts)
- Perceived lack of interest in partnering with your facility (locker slamming at 3 PM)
- CEO has no clue who you are
- Or the absence of any of the strengths

Threats:

- Large national companies who are always on the lookout for new practice opportunities
- Groups willing to enter your market at a substantial discount.

---

lowest quartile of patient satisfaction have a significantly worse patient outcome.[2] Organizations with higher patient satisfaction scores deliver higher quality care and also help the organization meet Value-Based Purchasing benchmarks. Higher patient satisfaction scores could be worth millions of dollars annually in Medicare payments to the organization. It is also important that each provider receives his or her quality scores for quality measures and for how those individual measures compare to the rest of the group. This will help drive quality and group promotion.

The Anesthesia Quality Institute or another Qualified Clinical Data Registry can help you analyze your outcomes as compared within the group as well as nationally. Benchmarking is a critical element for your group's quality improvement.

The PSH represents an opportunity for a group to demonstrate their serious intent to be a "partner" with the hospital or facility. Any attempt by a group to reduce the total cost of care will be viewed with admiration and enthusiasm by hospital administration.

Table 1
Elements of HCAHPS survey

Clinical Processes of Care	Patient Experience of Care (HCAHPS)	Clinical Care Outcomes	Safety of Care	Efficiency (Cost of Care Over 90-d Episode)
5%	25%	25%	20%	25%
• Immunization for influenza • Elective delivery before 39 d	• HCAHPS scores	• AMI mortality • Pneumonia mortality • Heart failure mortality	• Surgical site infection • Hospital-acquired conditions	• Cost of care (if above Medicare median, 0 points)

The HCAHPS score is composed of the following items: 1. communication with nurses; 2. communication with doctors; 3. responsiveness of hospital staff; 4. pain management; 5. communication about medicines; 6. cleanliness and quietness of hospital environment; 7. discharge information; 8. care transition; and 9. overall rating of hospital.
   Abbreviation: AMI, acute myocardial infarction; HCAHPS, Hospital Consumer Assessment of Healthcare Providers and Systems.

Threats: Large Groups and Discounted Groups

There is significant change in the health care threat landscape. This is exemplified by the trend for hospital consolidation (mergers), payer consolidation, anesthesia group consolidation, pressure from hospitals to employ their anesthesia groups, competition from large, well-capitalized anesthesia management companies (AMCs), and local and regional groups (Managed Services Organizations where groups aggregate for billing, contracting, and so forth, but stay financially separate). One of the advantages of an AMC to a hospital is that the AMC may be able to offer multiple service lines (eg, emergency medicine, neonatology, radiology) and cross-subsidize one specialty for another. With all the changes occurring, complacency cannot be tolerated. One must understand that health care organizations are under tremendous stress because of a myriad of factors. Part of this is due to shifting payer mix with an increase in governmental payers, a situation in which the hospital loses money on each patient cared for, and larger patient deductibles leading to worsening bad debt and pressure on the hospital's bottom line. Consolidation of insurers provide the insurers with market power to dictate prices (for example, in the Chicago area, Blue Cross has almost 70% of the commercial market and can almost dictate terms to hospitals), demands from medical staff for payment (call coverage, and so forth), competition from other facilities (eg, ambulatory surgery centers), and changing payment models with more at-risk contracts and Accountable Care Organizations, all compound the stresses in health care.

UNDERSTAND YOUR MARKET

You combine this SWOT analysis with a clear understanding of the market in which you practice to give you a competitive advantage. There are 2 types of competitive advantage: cost advantage (same product or service at a lower price) and differentiation advantage (better product or service at same price.) To find a competitive advantage, it is useful to know the forces that shape your industry.
   Michael Porter[3] described 5 competitive forces that shape an industry and can help you look at your business model and market and strategize for the future. These forces are known as Porter's Five Forces (**Fig. 4**):

1. Threat of new entrants
2. Bargaining power of suppliers

3. Bargaining power of customers (buyer power)
4. Jockeying for position among current competitors (competitive rivalry)
5. Threat of substitute products or services

In 2011, Scurlock and colleagues[4] described an academic anesthesia department needs assessment for creating a business strategy using Porter's 5. They stated "additional research in strategic decisions influencing anesthesia groups should focus on the threat of new entrants, bargaining power of suppliers, and the threat of substitute products or services."

Porter's 1: Threat of New Entrants

You can be replaced. Whatever your situation, please understand you can be replaced. Replacing an entire academic department is virtually impossible, but everyone else: you can be replaced. Never rely on contractual terms for protection from poor service or quality. There are too many examples of groups being replaced or forced to join more prepared and aggressive anesthesia groups who lobby a hospital for the anesthesia contract. These are the reasons your value proposition is critical.

Porter's 2: Bargaining Power of Suppliers

Does your group control the current anesthesia market? If so, you have supplier power. You are the sole source. As long as your value proposition remains strong and you constantly monitor your competitive advantage, you can remain the dominant supplier and exercise some control over the anesthesia market.

Porter's 3: Bargaining Power of Customers

Who is the customer? Ultimately, the customer is the patients, but initially hospitals, surgeons, private payers, and government entities. It is the balance of supplier and customer power that can be hard to maintain. If you constantly supply a superior product at a reasonable cost, you can maintain your level of influence. Hospital systems are powerful because they negotiate for system-wide contracts. Understanding who has

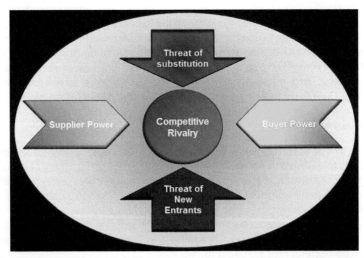

Fig. 4. Porter's 5 forces. (*From* Marketing theories—explaining Porter's five forces. Professional academy. Available at: https://www.professionalacademy.com/blogs-and-advice/marketing-theories—explaining-porters-five-forces. Accessed January 30, 2018; with permission.)

the bargaining power and how you can direct positive interest toward you and your group is an important skill.

Porter's 4: Competitive Rivalry

It is vital to understand that you are, or will be, in a competitive market. You should be using all the tools at your disposal to maintain a dominant position. National companies would love your practice, regardless of location. Positive cash flow is an enticing concept for investor groups.

Anesthesia management companies

The past 2 decades have seen a cataclysmic shift in the anesthesia market, with 8 large companies employing more than 20% of anesthesia providers compared with just a fraction 20 years ago. Some formations are the result of acquisitions, whereas others have been the result of an RFP being put out by their hospital resulting in an AMC taking over the contract for anesthesia services. The reasons for this change are 2-fold:

1. Growth of anesthesia services and
2. Potential for significant return on investment for the AMCs.

Some of the AMCs (MEDNAX and USAP) try to identify friendly merger and acquisition candidates, whereas others seek to aggressively take over hospital contracts at the expense of the extant anesthesia group. Other large multispecialty groups, such as Envision Healthcare, can step into anesthesia contracts as part of a broader hospital utilization of their services, such as emergency medicine, neonatology, and radiology. The anesthesia marketplace has seen a growth in large, well-managed, well-financed, national for-profit AMCs. They are playing a larger role in anesthesia practices. However, still slightly more than 50% of anesthesiologists work in groups of 50 or less, and 34% of physicians work in groups of 25 or less. **Table 2**[5] breaks down the number of anesthesia providers by group size.

Envision Healthcare and Mednax are examples of 2 large national AMCs. **Tables 3–5** look at their revenues, profits, and acquisitions over the period 2015 to 2016.

Fig. 5 is a graphical representation of 9 large national anesthesia practices and breaks those practices down those providers into physicians and Certified Registered Nurse Anesthetists (CRNAs).

Large AMCs may be able to negotiate higher reimbursement on anesthesia services either because of market power or expertise in negotiations. AMCs may also deliver economies of scale with respect to billing and other back office services. The other issue revolves around the willingness to become part of a larger organization. Despite

Table 2
Frequency distribution of physician anesthesiologists in groups

No. of Physician Anesthesiologists	No. of Groups	Total	Cumulative, %
300 or more	7	5394.8	16.1
≥100 & <300	30	4399.0	29.3
≥50 & <100	87	6063.7	47.4
≥25 & <50	178	6210.8	66.0
≥10 & <25	440	6665.3	86.0
≥5 & <10	453	3160.7	95.4
≥3 & <5	417	1534.6	100.0
Total groups of 3+	1612	33,428.9	—

the potential economies of scale and cross-subsidization of services, some large national companies are seeing some disturbing changes in the marketplace that has resulted in declining stock market values of almost 40% over the past year. These changes are related to a negative shift in payer mix (ie, more governmental payers), increasing labor costs (eg, CRNAs), performance bonuses not being achieved, and hospitals not always being pleased with staffing changes. Certain geographic markets have also been difficult for large national payers to enter (eg, Chicago). With these changes and declining profits and increasing costs, a slowing of the merger and acquisitions by these large national entities may be seen.

Envision Healthcare is an example of a large, national, multispecialty organization that employs more than 3000 anesthesia providers and operates in 48 states. This company serves more than 14 million patients annually, with nearly 13,000 affiliated clinicians at more than 1000 acute care hospitals in 48 states. In addition to anesthesia, Envision also provides services in emergency medicine, hospital medicine, acute care surgery, and radiology/teleradiology. Mednax is an example of another large, national multispecialty enterprise established in 101 hospitals, and 112 ambulatory surgery centers in 13 states. It includes pediatricians as well as radiologists. TeamHealth was founded in 1979 with the goal of providing emergency department administrative and staffing serves and is currently the largest national provider of hospital-based clinical outsourcing in multispecialties, including hospital and emergency medicine and anesthesia. It has a presence in 3400 civilian and military hospitals, clinics, and physician groups.

Porter's 5: Substitute Product or Service

Do competitors offer substitute products or services? Or *additional* products or services? Do you offer pediatric anesthesia because one of your venues wants to expand pediatric surgery? How about anesthesia for out of operating room (OR) locations? With whom are you competing and what do they offer that you do not? You need to be constantly surveilling your market, your practice, and your customers.

So now you know your group (SWOT) and your market (Porter's 5). What is next? Change the conversation. Change value to "results" and results to "outcomes." Michael Porter and Elizabeth Olmsted-Teisberg, in their seminal work, *Redefining Health Care*,[6,7] talk about "Creating Value Based Competition on Results." Thus, the value proposition becomes Outcomes/Cost. You must have data to show the superiority of your outcomes; outcomes differ among your customers, and you need to satisfy them all.

UNDERSTAND YOUR CUSTOMER

We know our customers are patients, surgeons, facilities, and payers. In our current market, our most important customer is the facility. Even if we keep everyone else

Table 3
Largest public companies with anesthesia practices (2015 operating data)

Company Name[a]	Total, $M	Anesthesia Related, %	Anesthesia Related, $M	Cases	Providers	Acquisitions
MEDNAX, Inc	2780	37.0	1029	1.53 M	2725	7
AmSurg Corp	2567	37.0	949	1.25 M	2900	6
Team Health	3597	11.0	396	n/a	400	11
Envision Healthcare	5448	4.7	255	n/a	n/a	n/a

Abbreviation: n/a, not applicable.
[a] Before merger of AmSurg and Envision Healthcare.

Table 4
Operating data Envision Healthcare and Mednax, 2015, 2016

	Operating Data				
	Envision Healthcare Corporation[a,b]			MEDNAX	
In Millions "$"		2015	2016	2015	2016
Net revenue		2567	3696	2779	3183
Income from operations		618	376	558	572
Net income		381	206	336	325
Profit margin (%)		14.8	5.6	12.1	10.2
Anesthesia-related revenue		1823	1072	1029	1241
Percentage revenue from anesthesia-related services		71.0	29.0	37.0	39.0

[a] 2017 consolidated financial statements: AmSurg for 3 mo ended March 31, 2016 and Envision Healthcare Corporation for 3 mo ended March 31, 2017.
[b] As of March 31, 2017.

happy, if the facility is not happy, we will be replaced; this is a simple fact. So, what does the facility CEO want from an anesthesia group? How do you go about putting this into action to achieve the best possible relationship with your hospital or Ambulatory Surgery Center (ASC) or any facility for that matter? *What are hospital CEOs looking for?*

They are looking for peace and quiet. *Satisfied silence* from the surgeons, patients, and OR staff.

Silence

Medicine is changing so fast both technologically and administratively that CEOs spend much of their time listening to problems and complaints. They do not need any negatives from a specialty that does not actually bring patients (and cash) to the hospital. In fact, this specialty is very costly, and for what?

Satisfied

A list follows of how to keep a CEO and hospital satisfied, thrilled to have you and your group provide anesthesia care, and seeing the real value in your value proposition (and remember absolute clinical excellence is assumed).

No Complaints About You

Show up on time: no case delays due to anesthesia issues. Be prepared; take a serious interest in and responsibility for the preoperative clinic, avoiding cancelations due to preventable anesthesia issues. Have one qualified group leader. No CEO wants to negotiate with multiple physicians for the same basic contract. No behavioral issues! Behavioral issues are the number one killer of anesthesia groups. If you have

Table 5
Summary of acquisitions (Envision Healthcare, MEDNAX), 2015-2016

Anesthesia-Related Physician Group Acquisitions			Anesthesia Professionals		
	2015	2016	Physician Anesthesiologists	CRNAs	Total
Envision Healthcare Corporation	6	8	1613	1472	3085
MEDNAX	7	8	1150	1575	2725

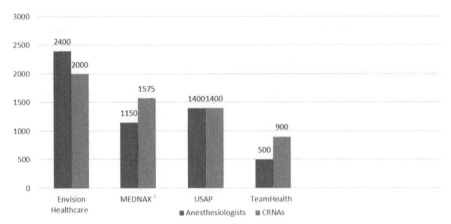

Fig. 5. Large national anesthesia entities, 2017.

a behavioral issue, fix it. Please, no bad mouthing anyone or anything publically in the OR.

Actually Help the Chief Executive Officer and Be a Partner with the Hospital

You must meet all regulatory requirements, have a patient satisfaction survey, and fix any problems it identifies. You must do NORA (non-OR anesthetizing) cases without whining, be fiscally responsible, be mindful of what things cost in the OR (drugs, supplies, and so forth). Use wisely. Help with OR efficiency. Move cases as necessary and do not hang on to cases because it benefits your personal income. Just get the schedule done to avoid overtime for everyone. Enthusiastically support reduced length of stay and patient experience. Support enhanced recovery after surgery (ERAS). Learn appropriate postoperative pain blocks and use them; patient satisfaction scores are the key to hospital payments from Medicare.

Reduce the Stipend

There is a clear trend toward stipend reduction nationally. When negotiating, be fact based and do not overshoot. Currently, approximately 80% of anesthesia groups receive some stipend from their hospital. This stipend is provided to ensure adequate coverage for hospital demands, which their patient volume and payer mix cannot support. There is constant pressure to reduce that stipend.

The truth is you do not WANT a stipend. *Imagine your value to your facility if you needed no stipend.* Through billing alone, you want to be able to recruit, retain, and support excellent anesthesiologists, anesthesia assistants (AAs), and CRNAs who are available whenever surgeons and proceduralists need your help. This is frequently impossible given the high percentage of government payers most hospitals have. However, there are actions you can take to save the hospital money, which effectively reduces the amount of money spent on an anesthesia group (they pay your "X", but you save them "Y", which makes their out-of-pocket costs X − Y, and so forth).

What can you do to save your hospital costs? This publication is full of ideas and their details, including improving OR efficiency, eliminating unnecessary laboratory/imaging costs, and early discharge through better postoperative pain management. Will the hospital help you with payer negotiations? The better the insurance payments, the less the hospital will need to pay in stipends. What about help with out-of-network patients? How can they help you help them reduce your stipend?

Take a Leadership Role in Your Facility

This is the opposite of do not cause trouble. You should cause good things to happen. Look for and find opportunities to champion perioperative initiatives that improve patient care and perioperative efficiency, such as the PSH. Be actively involved in your facilities' medical staff committees, such as OR management, pharmacy and therapeutics, quality improvement, and the medical executive committee.

What are our other customers looking for?

- Surgeons: very straightforward: start cases on time. Make sure their patients are satisfied and comfortable, do not remember the surgery, and don't move (not necessarily in that order)!
- Insurance companies: low-cost, high patient satisfaction (no complaints). To negotiate with anyone, remember to have data: the more the better, and local standards, community standards, and national standards, and what makes you special.
- Government: Meet all the "standards" set by Centers for Medicare and Medicaid Services and control cost control. Look at the Merit-based Incentive Payment System (MIPS) part of the new Medicare Access and CHIP Reauthorization Act (MACRA) law. That lays out exactly what the government wants.
- Patients: be a member of my insurance network, "help me, don't hurt me," be nice to me, control my pain, control my postoperative nausea and vomiting, help me recover faster (peripheral nerve blocks).

Finally, what is your value proposition? What do you bring to the table? Divide your value into 3 categories: clinical, nonclinical, and cost.

Clinical

Start with the PSH. Can you do at least some parts of this concept?

The PSH is a patient-centered, physician-led, interdisciplinary, and team-based system of coordinated care (**Fig. 6**). The PSH spans the entire surgical episode from the decision of the need of an invasive procedure: surgical, diagnostic, or therapeutic, to discharge and beyond. It is designed to achieve the triple aim of improving health, improving the delivery of health care, and reducing the cost of care.

The current landscape of surgical care is highly variable and fragmented. It finds physicians working in silos, in a very disjointed and uncoordinated manner, at high cost, with unnecessary or prolonged skilled nursing facility stays. It also has many episodes of delays and efficiencies, long length of stays, patients who do not feel they are listened to, and high complications and outcomes that are less than optimal.

The PSH is closely aligned with the shift in medicine from volume to cost, and the PSH care model has shown a reduction in complications, eliminates silos and the fragmented care process, shortens length of stay, assures appropriate cost-effective care after discharge, and reduces readmissions. The PSH is physician-led (a surgeon, anesthesiologist, or other physician) system of comprehensive care that provides an anesthesia group the opportunity to be front and center with care redesign processes, improved outcomes, and lower costs to health care institutions.

Are you indeed clinically excellent? Do you have data to show your outcomes are better than anyone else? Are you surveying and asking your patients, surgeons, and

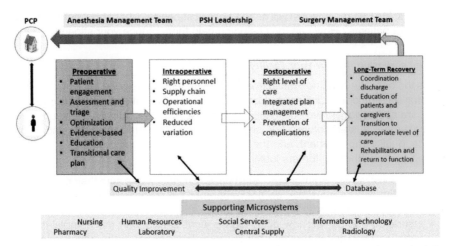

Fig. 6. The 4 phases of care under the PSH. (*Courtesy of* American Society of Anesthesiologists, Schaumburg, IL.)

hospital if they are satisfied with your performance, and working on any deficiencies, perceived or otherwise? Remember perception is reality until proved otherwise (facts, data!!).

Do you meet all regulatory requirements? Are you concerned with stopping surgical site infections? Are you skilled at peripheral nerve blocks? Facile with ultrasound? List your competitors.

Nonclinical

It is essential that your department has *a strong core leadership* group and that the individual who is chosen to lead the group is the right person for the job. He or she must have the tools to lead and deal with hospital administration, not simply because of tenure with the group or likeability. It is also important that the group acts as one and does not air its dirty laundry in public. It is fine to have constructive dissent in the group, but when dealing with others, the group must be seen as speaking with one voice and working off of one playbook. The group needs to give leadership, and those serving on hospital committees, time and the financial backing to help promote the group. This cannot be precisely quantified in billing units but is in many ways more valuable than delivering great care, which is always considered the baseline.

It is vital that groups deal with disruptive providers and take steps to prevent those disruptors from sabotaging all the other good things the group does. The fastest way for a group to lose credibility with administration is the failure to deal with the underperforming provider (whether in quality or personality). It is important that there are policies and codes of conduct (enforced uniformly) in places that address these issues and also that disruptive behavior is documented and acted on with either legal counsel or human resources (if the group is large enough or part of a multispecialty or hospital-owned group). Small- to medium-size groups must have agreed upon policies because it can be difficult to deal with the disruptive or underperforming member, especially if that member is an equal partner in the group structure.

Costs

Hospitals hate stipends, but with proper negotiation, they can understand the business concept that you need to purchase quality service if the outside market cannot meet the needs. Negotiation is a complex topic and cannot be addressed easily and requires both training and expertise in this area. Often it is best to bring in an outside negotiator or consultant to advocate for the group. It is important to also understand the needs of the hospital (as health care organizations are facing tremendous cost pressures and other physician groups are also approaching the hospital for their own support) and also to clarify in your thought processes the important issues that face your group. Negotiations should be seen as a win-win, rather than a one-off, as it is hoped the relationship with the hospital or health care organization is a long-term one. Rather than an adversarial relationship, a mutually beneficial partnership should be sought. Anesthesia groups should look to be a proactive partner with the hospital and seek ways to enhance the way the organization looks at you with new initiatives (ERAS, pain management, reducing patient length of stay).

SUMMARY

Your group's Value Proposition is crucial to developing a competitive advantage in your market. It helps others understand and appreciate your value, and it helps your group understand what is expected of them to meet the high levels of clinical and nonclinical performance you have set for your group.

By developing your value proposition, you also develop a keen understanding of your market (Porter's 5) as well as your own internal workings (SWOT Analysis). You will know your competitors and how they differ from you and what they offer and what you need to compete.

You know what you can offer to your customers because you also develop a keen understanding of them as well as what makes you special. You will have collected data about quality outcomes and patient satisfaction. You will fully understand the cost of your services and the pressure the hospital is under to reduce costs.

The Value Proposition gives you something tangible when you go to negotiate with any of your customers. We know our value, but often communicate it poorly. Now is the time to fix that and make sure all our customers know how much value we bring to our relationships.

REFERENCES

1. Available at: https://www.mckinsey.com/business-functions/strategy-and-corporate-finance/our-insights/delivering-value-to-customers.
2. Tsai TC, Orav JE, Jha A. Patient satisfaction and quality of surgical care in US hospital. Ann Surg 2015;261:2–8.
3. Porter M. How competitive forces shape strategy. Harv Bus Rev 1979;59:137–45.
4. Scurlock C, Dexter F, Reich DL, et al. Needs assessment for business strategies of anesthesiology groups' practices. Anesth Analg 2011;113:170–4.
5. 2016 Physician Compare National Downloadable File. Available at: https://data.medicare.gov/Physician-Compare/Physician-Compare-National-Downloadable-File/mj5m-pzi6/data. Accessed August, 2017.
6. Porter M, Olmsted-Teisberg E. Redefining healthcare: creating value-based competition on results. Boston (MA): Harvard Business Review Press; 2006.
7. MEDNAX. Health Solutions Partner. Available at: https://www.mednax.com/hospitals/solutions/.

Bundled Payments and Hidden Costs

Stanley W. Stead, MD, MBA, FASA[a],*, Sharon K. Merrick, MS, CCS-P[b]

KEYWORDS

- Bundled payment • Episodes of care • Health care reform • Total joint replacement

KEY POINTS

- In a fee-for-service environment, anesthesiologists are paid for the volume of services billed, with little relation to the cost of delivering the services.
- Bundled payments are a set fee for an episode of care, including all anesthesia, pain medicine, and related services for the surgical episode and a period of time thereafter procedure to cover complications and redo procedures.
- When calculating a bundled payment, all the services typically used by a patient must be counted when calculating both the costs and expected payment.

INTRODUCTION

New health care financing models are challenging traditional fee for service. "Medicare is moving toward an episode-based reimbursement system combining hospital and physician payment, which is expected to reduce government outlays."[1] Accountable care organizations are being touted as the new model for payment of medical services. Originally described by Elliot Fisher, MD, MPH, a Dartmouth researcher, the key concepts were the following:

1. Providers should become accountable for the overall quality and cost of care for the populations they serve.
2. Provider incomes must be decoupled from volume and intensity of services performed; pay should reflect better value, improved outcomes, better quality and reduced costs.
3. The accountable care organization should adopt fully transparent and meaningful performance measures on both quality and cost. This is necessary to overcome patient resistance. Also, reliable risk-adjusted measures of overall costs are a required element so as to measure impact of care changes at the local level.

Disclosures: The authors have nothing to disclose.
[a] Stead Health Group, Inc, 4819 Andasol Avenue, Suite 100, Encino, CA 91316, USA; [b] American Society of Anesthesiologists, Inc, 905 16th Street, Northwest, Suite 400, Washington, DC 20006, USA
* Corresponding author.
E-mail address: Stan.Stead@Stead-Group.com

Anesthesiology Clin 36 (2018) 241–258
https://doi.org/10.1016/j.anclin.2018.01.005   anesthesiology.theclinics.com
1932-2275/18/© 2018 Elsevier Inc. All rights reserved.

Abbreviations	
CF	Conversion factor
CMS	Centers for Medicare & Medicaid Services
CPT	Current Procedural Terminology
ICD-9-CM	International Classification of Diseases, 9th Edition, Clinical Modification
ICD-10-CM	International Classification of Diseases, 10th Edition, Clinical Modification
PACU	Postanesthesia care unit
TDABC	Time-driven activity-based costing

Although payment for primary care services is focused on periodic service to keep patients healthy (medical home), it is clear that different payments will be necessary for those providing care when the patients are no longer healthy. In the case of surgical care, much work in recent years has focused on payments surgical episodes. The Centers for Medicare & Medicaid Services (CMS) have done a number of demonstration projects for some cardiovascular and orthopedic procedures. Currently, CMS has ongoing bundled payments for care improvement initiative in which a single, fixed amount is paid and shared by hospitals and physicians who provide the care. Bundled payments for care improvement payment distribution structures can vary based on the model. The Medicare Access and CHIP Reauthorization Act takes this to another level, with all Medicare payment predicated on quality and costs of care. Under the Medicare Access and CHIP Reauthorization Act, considerable pressure is being applied to providers and hospitals to move toward alternative payment models. Key component in alternative payment models are bundled payments, with bonus payments for reducing costs and financial penalties for those who do not.

How can an anesthesia practice determine its costs and the income necessary to cover its services in such a system? It is important to understand our current economic model and how to apply the information from our practices in formulating an episode-based fee. Today, deteriorating payer mix and increased coverage demands without the matching delivery of clinical services have driven down payments and, therefore, income. Anesthesiologists are reasonably concerned about a new payment model that adds more financial risk to their practice.

In this article, we provide background on current billing, cost, and revenue processes and show how to use these data to determine the right bundled payment that the group needs to continue to be successful. The checklist in **Box 1** should guide your development of a bundled payment.

Box 1
Checklist for determining bundled payments

Which conditions will the bundled payments be applied?

What services should be included in the bundled payment?

Which providers are included, and how is their participation determined?

How should payments be set?

What is the scope or timeframe of the bundle?

Can the bundled payment be risk adjusted?

What data need to be available to monitor and administer the practice's costs and payments?

ANESTHESIA ECONOMICS 101 (1992 TO 2016)

In the fee-for-service payment model, where volume drives income, successful anesthesia practices maximize the unit production, conversion factor (CF) rate, and account collection. Anesthesia costs are composed of physician salary, practice expenses, and professional liability. Because the salary was what remained after practice expense and professional liability were paid, successful practices minimized their overall costs by minimizing the billing costs, consolidating the anesthetizing locations, and minimizing the administrative costs. In many markets, anesthesia costs were covered by income from clinical activities.

In this era, the emphasis was on capturing all charges for services provided and submitting accurate and timely claims. Key tools included the Current Procedural Terminology (CPT) and the *International Classification of Diseases*, 9th Edition, Clinical Modification (ICD-9-CM)/*International Classification of Diseases*, 10th Edition, Clinical Modification (ICD-10-CM) code sets along with resources specific to anesthesia such as the American Society of Anesthesiologists Relative Value Guide and CROSSWALK.

Quality of care entered the scene in 2007 with the Physician Voluntary Reporting Program, which evolved into the Physician Quality Reporting Initiative, and then into the Physician Quality Reporting System. These quality reporting programs initially provided for upward payment adjustments for reporting and then moved into downward adjustment for not reporting. Medicare payments were also impacted (positively or negatively) at the group or Taxpayer Identification Number level by the value-based payment modifier.

Anesthesia Revenue

Anesthesia services are typically paid according to "base + time." Anesthesia services described by a CPT code are assigned a base unit value that corresponds with the intensity and complexity of the care. It includes the usual preoperative and postoperative visits, administration of fluids and/or blood products, and the interpretation of noninvasive monitoring. It does not include the placement of invasive monitoring devices such as central venous lines or procedures performed for postoperative pain control. Time is the time spent providing anesthesia care. It starts when the anesthesiologist begins to prepare the patient for anesthesia care in the operating room or an equivalent area and ends when the patient is placed under the care of the postanesthesia care unit (PACU).[2] There are physical status modifiers that may apply for patients who are not Medicare beneficiaries. Base and time units added together, along with applicable modifiers, are multiplied by a CF to determine the charge.

Unlike surgery, which may report and receive payment for multiple procedures performed on a patient during a single session, only one anesthesia procedure may be reported during a single surgical session. The anesthesia procedure reported should be the most complex anesthetic service; however, the cumulative time for all the surgical procedures is reported.

Nonanesthesia services are exceptions to this general rule. Examples are placement of invasive monitoring lines, which is billed separately, and postoperative pain management procedures that may be separately reported under specific circumstances. An important feature of nonanesthesia services that is not applicable to anesthesia is a global period. The payment for these nonanesthesia services may include only the care provided on the day of the procedure or it may include all associated care for a period of days after the procedure. For example, interlaminar epidural injections (CPT codes 62320–62327) have a 0-day global period. Any medically necessary follow-up care subsequent to the date of the injection is reported separately. In contrast, paravertebral facet joint ablation (CPT codes 64633–64635) have a 10-day global period. The payment includes the work on the day of the procedure and all follow-up care over the next 10 days. That follow-up care is not reported separately. This coding could be viewed as a procedure-specific bundle.

Anesthesia Costs

A practice cannot control its costs without understanding what those costs are. Current costing methodology is based on direct expense assignment (percent of charge for hospital and work; relative value units for a professional service) with an allocation for indirect costs. Frequently, we see practices simply looking at the provider costs. What is the cost of an anesthesiologist? One method totals the median compensation of an anesthesiologist with the practice and professional liability costs and divides by the hours of care provided. We will assume that the typical private anesthesiologist receives $411,000 in professional compensation representing 44 weeks worked per year, 55 hours per week, or 2420 hours per year.[3] For this discussion, we will use Medicare's determination that professional compensation is 78.3% of the practice income,[4] giving us $524,900 of practice income per anesthesiologist. Practice income needs to be $217 per hour, corresponding with an hourly wage of $170 per our. To break even, the anesthesia practice needs to collect more than $217 per hour, because some of the clinical time is spent in uncompensated activities, or simply waiting. In a busy practice, 70% of the clinical time is compensated, indicating that practice income needs to be ($217/0.70) $310 per hour or $5.17 per minute. Similar calculations can be done for nurse anesthetists and anesthesiologist assistants.

When practice is in a care team model, the relative costs depend greatly on the model, and the average ratio of physicians to anesthesia provider. Staffing costs range between 75% and 130% of an anesthesiologist practicing alone.[3]

Another method for determining costs is time-driven activity-based costing (TDABC).[5,6] TDABC assigns costs for each resource consumed in providing a clinical service based on the price paid for that resource and the quantity of that resource used. TDABC allows the assignment of cost rates, along with the capacity rates for each of the resources. TDABC illuminates inefficiencies and provides a method to measure the change in costs resulting from a change in process. TDABC is very situation specific. The TDABC model requires defining a care blueprint, process maps for each activity in the patient care delivery, identification of resources needed at each step, and time estimates for each process step. Using TDABC methodology, the costs of an anesthesiologist in total joint replacement programs was estimated at $5.80 per minute.[7]

For the remaining discussion, we assume an anesthesiologist costs $300 per hour, or $5 per minute.

ANESTHESIA ECONOMICS 201 (2017 AND BEYOND?)

In the future, anesthesia practices may need or want to participate in acute care episode payment models. Episode payments are designed to compensate for the average or typical costs incurred during the entire period of care. To be sure you cover all your costs, you need to understand your patient demographics, your practice parameters, your payer's contribution to your practice, practice collections, and practice costs (**Fig. 1**). It is important to define the episode of care. It can be as short as the surgical admission or as long as the surgical global period. In the case of total joint

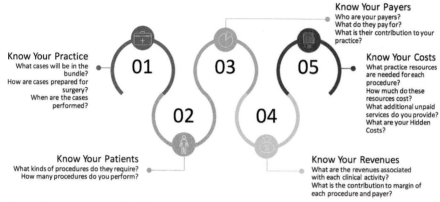

Know Your Payers
Who are your payers?
What do they pay for?
What is their contribution to your practice?

Know Your Practice
What cases will be in the bundle?
How are cases prepared for surgery?
When are the cases performed?

01   **03**   **05**

02   **04**

Know Your Costs
What practice resources are needed for each procedure?
How much do these resources cost?
What additional unpaid services do you provide?
What are your Hidden Costs?

Know Your Patients
What kinds of procedures do they require?
How many procedures do you perform?

Know Your Revenues
What are the revenues associated with each clinical activity?
What is the contribution to margin of each procedure and payer?

Fig. 1. Five step process for determining a bundled payment.

replacement, because of the high complication rate associated with knee replacement, payers may seek a rate for the 90-day surgical global period.

Table 1 illustrates how Medicare determines the allowed amount for anesthesia care of a hip replacement. For simplicity, a Medicare anesthesia CF of $22 per unit ($22.1887) was used.

The Medicare allowed amount is $365.20. After the deductible is met, Medicare pays 80% of the allowed amount and the patient (or secondary insurance) is responsible for the 20% balance. Although anesthesia intraservice time is carefully accounted for and paid, some additional time is required to provide a complete anesthesia service. For total joints, each case requires preoperative evaluation (20 minutes), time in the PACU (10 minutes), time for evaluating the recovery from anesthesia (10 minutes) and perhaps pain medicine management (5 minutes), yielding an additional 45 minutes per case that is not directly captured or reportable in your claims. Assuming that the preoperative visit took 20 minutes, PACU care an additional 20 minutes, and the case time is 129 minutes, the total time is 169 minutes. At a cost of $5 per minute, the anesthesiologist cost for this case is $845. The total payment received was $365.20, assuming the 20% patient copayment was made. Overall the practice loses an average of $480 per case. How is this possible?

Medicare pays disproportionally less for anesthesia than it does for other specialties. In the 2007 US Government Accountability Office report, Medicare Physician

Table 1
Medicare calculation for anesthesia payment of joint replacement

Anesthesia CPT Code	01214 - Anesthesia for Hip Arthroplasty	01402 - Anesthesia for Knee Arthroplasty
Base units	8	7
Anesthesia time (min)	129	123
Time units	8.6	8.2
Base units + time units	16.6	15.2
Conversion factor (sample)	$22	$22
(Base + time) × conversion factor	$365.20	$334.40

Payments: Medicare and Private Payment Differences for Anesthesia Services, anesthesiologists were paid only 33% of commercial rates[8]:

[The US Government Accountability Office] found that in 2004 average Medicare payments for a set of seven anesthesia services provided by anesthesiologists alone were 67 percent lower than average private insurance payments in 41 Medicare payment localities—geographic areas established by CMS to account for geographic variations in the relative costs of providing physician services.

A bundled payment based on Medicare rate payments would not compensate for the practice costs.

To determine an anesthesia case rate for hip and knee replacements, a group might consider several options. One method uses current collections and sets a case rate based on a weighted average. A group would need to know the minimum CF it must have to cover its costs, as well as the number of anesthetics it provides for these cases for a given time span and the average anesthesia time. Some groups may propose a case rate based on the commercial CF.

Table 2 shows the typical distribution of cases in a private practice. In this initial example, only the cases reported with 3 anesthesia CPT codes were used in the calculation: Anesthesia for Total Knee Arthroplasty (CPT Code 01402), Anesthesia for Total Hip Arthroplasty (01214) and Anesthesia for Revision of Total Hip Arthroplasty (01215). Some total joints were under coded as Anesthesia for Open Procedures involving Hip Joint (01210). In 2017, Medicare paid approximately $22 per unit and private payers commercial contracts ranged from $71 to $83 per unit.[9] We use a commercial CF of $75 per unit.

Using the formula of (base + time) × CF:

Hips: $(8 + 122/15) \times \$75 = \$1223$

Revised hips: $(10 + 175/15) \times \$75 = \$1628$

Knees: $(7 + 123/15) \times \$75 = \$1140$

Table 2
Initial look: total joint replacement surgical cases

Procedures	Medicare Cases (n)	Commercial Cases (n)	Total Cases (N)	Medicare Average Payment ($)	Commercial Average Payment ($)	Average Payment ($)	Average Time (min)
01214 - Anesthesia for hip arthroplasty	74	48	122	359	1223	698	129
01215 - Anesthesia for revision hip repair	6	4	10	477	1628	937	202
01402 - Anesthesia for knee arthroplasty	92	97	189	334	1140	748	124
Average	172	149	321	350	1180	735	129

If the case rate is the weighted average of hips and knees:

$$(48 \times \$1223) + (4 \times \$1628) + (97 \times \$1140)/(48 + 4 + 97) = \$1180$$

The practice costs would be the sum of the weighted average of hip, revised hip, and knee intraservice times (125 min) and preservice and postservice times listed above (40 min), 165 minutes or $825. The difference between the weighted average payment of $1180 yields a profit of $354 per commercial case. Hopefully, this difference would cover the losses in Medicare and other payers with low CFs.

However, if you accept this simple analysis, you will lose money! This basic analysis has not taken into account the additional procedures associated with the cases, such as invasive monitoring, postoperative pain management, and any additional anesthesia procedures that may be associated with complications or other requirements within the global period of the bundled payment.

To properly understand your practice's revenues and costs, you need to use your practice management data. For the remainder of this article, we use a sample dataset that was derived from an actual practice. However, the payment and charge data have been modified to reflect current CMS and American Society of Anesthesiologists mean CF survey data.[9]

Assumptions

To perform these calculations, the data must be stored in a way that the group can access it and use it. At a minimum, an anesthesia group should have a year's worth of billing and practice data in a tool that allows manipulation of the data (such as Excel or Access). The dataset must include a robust number of elements, including but not limited to:

Patient demographics
- Name
- Hospital ID number
- Hospital encounter number
- Gender
- Date of birth

Payer information
- Primary payer and contractual allowance
- Secondary payer and contractual allowance
- Patient copayment

Practice information
- All services provided during a typical surgical episode
- Units generated
- Anesthesia time
- Cost of resources required to provide care
- Other overhead expenses

Using Your Practice Data

Let's assume that your hospital approaches your practice to identify a bundled payment for total joints (hips and knees) for non-Medicare patients. Your hospital has been successfully participating in the CMS Comprehensive Care for Joint Replacement Model and, although the hospital was receiving bundled payments, you were paid Medicare rates for all the cases. With your checklist in hand (see **Box 1**), from the discussions you determine the following requirements:

- Conditions: Total hip replacement, revision of total hip replacement, total knee replacement and revision of total knee replacement.
- Services from anesthesia: Operative anesthesia, pain management during hospitalization.
- Providers: Physician anesthesiologists, nurse anesthetists, anesthesiologist's assistants, pain medicine physicians.
- Payment: Single fee, paid at the end of the 90 days after discharge.
- Scope and timeframe of the bundle: At this time, the hospital wants to include all payers, but will consider different rates for Medicare and commercial. The timeframe is 3 days before procedure and 90 days after discharge, to include all complications and rework.
- Risk adjustment: None.
- Data: Hospital will notify practice of all patients participating in the bundled payment. Updates will be provided weekly. The hospital notes that 369 cases were performed in the previous calendar year that would qualify.

You search your practice billing and determine that you have performed a total of 321 total joint cases in the previous year. In this example, the average practice total joint payment is $700. This is significantly lower than the commercial rate, which would yield $1183. However, based on clinical time, the practice costs are $877 per case. On average, the practice is losing $177 per case. You decide to propose a bundled case price of $877, based on the average time and payment. However, when presented to the hospital, they note that your data seem to be missing some of the patients. The number of cases listed does not match what the surgeons are reporting in the same period.

A Review of your practice data shows that only CPT codes Anesthesia for Total Knee Arthroplasty (CPT code 01402), Anesthesia for Total Hip Arthroplasty (01214), and Anesthesia for Revision of Total Hip Arthroplasty (01215) were used in the calculation. Some total joints were under coded as Anesthesia for Open Procedures involving Hip Joint (01210) or Anesthesia for Open Procedures involving Upper Two-Thirds of Femur (01230). To correctly determine the case frequency, it is useful to look at all the surgical cases by ICD-10 diagnosis codes and, if you have the data, the surgical CPT code. We have provided a list of all the procedures that were done on patients who would be classified as total joints during the entire 90-day global period (**Table 3**). Based on this additional information, the additional total joint cases were reassigned to 1 of the 3 categories (**Table 4**).

In addition, payment is often reported in aggregate form. It is important to separate the cases by payer. When the correct data are retrieved and grouped into Medicare and commercial payers, it again confirms that Medicare is only paying at about 33% of the commercial rate.

On average, $1205 is the case payment rate for commercial payers (see **Table 4**), but this does not cover all the services the patient may receive. We observe that some patients had preoperative consults weeks before their surgery and independent of the preoperative evaluation. Further, some patients were identified as American Society of Anesthesiologists physical status 3 or greater, some required invasive monitoring, and some received postoperative acute pain management. Finally, some patients required additional related procedures during the surgical global period.

A group must also include the nonanesthesia services it provides as part of the surgical episode. Because these services are reported using the Resource-Based

Table 3
Procedures reported with total joint replacements by anesthesiologists

CPT Code	Brief Description	CPT Procedures Descriptors
00400	Anesthesia for skin procedures	Anesthesia for procedures on the integumentary system on the extremities, anterior trunk and perineum; not otherwise specified
01210	Anesthesia for hip joint surgery	Anesthesia for open procedures involving hip joint; not otherwise specified
01214	Anesthesia for hip arthroplasty	Anesthesia for open procedures involving hip joint; total hip arthroplasty
01215	Anesthesia for revision hip repair	Anesthesia for open procedures involving the hip joint; revision of total hip arthroplasty
01220	Anesthesia for closed procedure on femur	Anesthesia for all closed procedures involving upper two-thirds of the femur
01230	Anesthesia for open surgery on femur	Anesthesia for open procedures involving the upper two-thirds of femur; not otherwise specified
01270	Anesthesia for upper leg artery surgery	Anesthesia for procedures involving arteries of the upper leg, including bypass graft; not otherwise specified
01360	Anesthesia for lower femur surgery	Anesthesia for all open procedures on the lower one-third of the femur
01380	Anesthesia for knee joint closed procedure	Anesthesia for all closed procedures on the knee joint
01392	Anesthesia for knee area surgery	Anesthesia for all open procedures on the upper ends of the tibia, fibula, and/or patella
01400	Anesthesia for knee joint surgery	Anesthesia for open or surgical arthroscopic procedures on the knee joint; not otherwise specified
01402	Anesthesia for knee arthroplasty	Anesthesia for open or surgical arthroscopic procedures on the knee joint; total knee arthroplasty
01480	Anesthesia for lower leg surgery	Anesthesia for open procedures on bones of the lower leg, ankle, and foot; not otherwise specified
01996	Daily hospital management of drug infusion	Daily hospital management of epidural or subarachnoid continuous drug administration
36556	Insertion CVC	Insertion of a nontunneled centrally inserted central venous catheter; age ≥ 5 y
36620	Insert A-line	Arterial catheterization or cannulation for sampling, monitoring or transfusion (separate procedure); percutaneous
62322	Single-shot lumbar interlaminar epidural	Injection(s) of diagnostic or therapeutic substance(s) (eg, anesthetic, antispasmodic, opioid, steroid, other solution), not including neurolytic substances, including needle or catheter placement, interlaminar epidural or subarachnoid, lumbar or sacral (caudal); without imaging guidance

(continued on next page)

Table 3
(continued)

CPT Code	Brief Description	CPT Procedures Descriptors
62326	Lumbar interlaminar epidural catheter	Injection(s), including indwelling catheter placement, continuous infusion or intermittent bolus, of diagnostic or therapeutic substance(s) (eg, anesthetic, antispasmodic, opioid, steroid, other solution), not including neurolytic substances, interlaminar epidural or subarachnoid, lumbar or sacral (caudal); without imaging guidance
64447	Single-shot femoral nerve block	Injection, anesthetic agent; femoral nerve, single
64448	Continuous femoral nerve block	Injection, anesthetic agent; femoral nerve, continuous infusion by catheter (including catheter placement)
64449	Continuous lumbar plexus catheter	Injection, anesthetic agent; lumbar plexus, posterior approach, continuous infusion by catheter (including catheter placement)
99100	Anesthesia for extreme age	Anesthesia for patient of extreme age, <1 y and >70 y (list separately in addition to code for primary anesthesia procedure)
99140	Emergency anesthesia	Anesthesia complicated by emergency conditions (specify) (list separately in addition to code for primary anesthesia procedure)

Current Procedural Terminology (CPT) is a list of descriptive terms and identifying numeric codes maintained by the American Medical Association for medical services and procedures that are provided by physicians and health care professionals.

Abbreviations: A-line, arterial line; CVC, central venous catheter.

Courtesy of American Medical Association (AMA), Chicago, IL; with permission.

Table 4
Updated total joint cases

Anesthesia Procedures for Total Joint Replacement	Medicare Cases (n)	Commercial Cases (n)	Total Cases (N)	Medicare Average Payment ($)	Commercial Average Payment ($)	Average Payment ($)	Average Time (min)
01214 - Anesthesia for hip arthroplasty	85	52	137	365	1245	700	129
01215 - Anesthesia for revision hip repair	8	6	14	517	1763	1051	202
01402 - Anesthesia for knee arthroplasty	115	95	210	337	1148	704	124
Average	208	153	361	355	1205	715	129

Relative Value Scale payment system, we use the Medicare payment for the service, assuming the practice places a central venous line in 10% of these patients, CPT code 36556:

Medicare payment is 3.48 relative value units at $36 = $125

$$([85 + 8 + 115] \times 10\%) \times \$125 = \$2600$$

Or an average of $125 \times 10\% = \$12.50$ per case

While doing the above analysis, your colleagues point out that there are a number of services that patients are receiving. For each patient who received anesthesia services for joint replacement, you extract all the services they received during the global period, or 90 days from the date of discharge and 3 days before the surgery.

You analyze all the charges for patients who received total joint replacement and separate the commercial payers from Medicare. We then calculate the frequency of other CPT codes reported with the total joint replacement (**Table 5**). Your practice has been tracking the amount of time each invasive monitor or block is taking, so

Table 5
Charge frequency of other CPT codes, reported with all total joint replacement episodes

CPT Procedures Reported with Total Joints	Average Time (min)	Commercial Payers			Medicare		
		Total Hip	Revised Total Hip	Total Knee	Total Hip	Revised Total Hip	Total Knee
01996 Daily hospital management of drug infusion	15	0	0	33	0	0	41
36556 Insertion CVC	15	0	0	0	18	2	1
36620 - Insert A-line	10	1	1	1	4	0	3
62322 - Single-shot lumbar interlaminar epidural	11	34	2	52	47	3	59
62326 - Lumbar interlaminar epidural catheter	15	1	0	0	0	0	1
64447 - Single-shot femoral nerve block	15	0	0	14	0	0	28
64448 - Continuous femoral nerve block	15	0	0	25	0	0	31
64449 - Continuous lumbar plexus catheter	—	0	0	0	1	0	0
99100 - Anesthesia for extreme age	0	4	0	6	67	0	64
99140 - Emergency anesthesia	0	1	5	7	4	0	4
Total Additional Procedures	—	41	8	105	141	5	191
Total additional time (min)	—	399	32	1662	827	63	2209
Average additional time (min)	—	10	4	12	6	13	10

Abbreviations: A-line, arterial line; CPT, Current Procedural Terminology.

the total additional minutes these procedures take, along with the average additional time per total joint replacement case is calculated. From that you can estimate the time each procedure takes. Similarly, we determine the average payment per procedure for the total joint patients in **Table 6**.

Bundling calculations should also include the payments for additional CPT codes billed for total joint replacement. The total case rate would reflect the sum of the payment for the anesthesia CPT codes and the additional CPT codes reported.

Anesthesia Economic Modeling

Actuarial science analyzes the rates of disability, morbidity, mortality, fertility, and other contingencies. The effects of consumer choice, the geographic distribution of the use of medical services and procedures, and the use of drugs and therapies, are also of great importance. These factors underlay the development of the resource-based relative value scale.

Practices need to use economic modeling similar to what actuaries use. For this analysis, we assumed the historical frequency and type of surgical cases accurately represents the case frequency and type of the future population. We also assumed a constant surgical case rate. For the purposes of the analysis:

- Patient selection remains the same;
- Surgical approach/procedure remains the same;
- Complication rates from the surgical cases remains the same;

Table 6
Average payments per case for CPT codes reported with total joint replacement

CPT Procedures Reported with Total Joints	Commercial Payers ($)			Medicare ($)		
	Total Hip	Revised Total Hip	Total Knee	Total Hip	Revised Total Hip	Total Knee
01996 Daily hospital management of drug infusion	—	—	78	—	—	24
36556 Insertion CVC	—	—	—	27	31	1
36620 - Insert A-line	2	15	1	2	—	1
62322 - Single-shot lumbar interlaminar epidural	99	51	83	50	34	47
62326 - Lumbar interlaminar epidural catheter	3	—	—	—	—	1
64447 - Single-shot femoral nerve block	—	—	17	—	—	17
64448 - Continuous femoral nerve block	—	—	32	—	—	20
64449 - Continuous lumbar plexus catheter	—	—	—	1	—	—
99100 - Anesthesia for extreme age	6	—	5	—	—	—
99140 - Emergency anesthesia	3	125	11	—	—	—
Average payment	113	190	227	80	65	110

Abbreviations: A-line, arterial line; CPT, Current Procedural Terminology.

- Treatment modalities that may result in anesthesia services remains unchanged; and
- Complication rates from the anesthetic management and type of anesthetic is unchanged.

The surgical procedures experienced by the patients who received total joint replacement within 90 days of the initial joint replacement were selected. The frequency associated with additional anesthesia services required during the 90-day episode is summarized in **Table 7**. In addition, the average additional minutes for these cases was determined.

Based on the practice data, 5.8% to 16.7% of the commercial total joints require additional surgery during the global period, which represents $ to -$203, or an average

Table 7
Charge frequency of anesthesia for additional surgical services in total joint replacement 90-day global period

Additional Anesthesia Procedures Reported During Global Period	Commercial Payers			Medicare		
	Total Hip	Revised Total Hip	Total Knee	Total Hip	Revised Total Hip	Total Knee
00400 - Anesthesia for skin procedures	—	—	—	1	—	—
01210 - Anesthesia for hip joint surgery	1	—	—	2	—	—
01214 - Anesthesia for hip arthroplasty	—	—	1	—	—	—
01215 - Anesthesia for revise hip repair	—	—	1	—	—	—
01220 - Anesthesia for closed procedure on femur	—	1	—	1	—	—
01230 - Anesthesia for open surgery on femur	1	—	5	2	—	—
01270 - Anesthesia for upper leg artery surgery	—	—	—	—	—	2
01360 - Anesthesia for lower femur surgery	—	—	2	—	—	2
01380 - Anesthesia for knee joint closed procedure	—	—	3	—	—	—
01392 - Anesthesia for knee area surgery	—	—	1	—	—	—
01400 - Anesthesia for knee joint surgery	—	—	—	—	—	1
01402 - Anesthesia for knee arthroplasty	1	—	1	—	—	1
01480 - Anesthesia for lower leg surgery	—	—	1	1	—	2
Additional procedures	3	1	15	7	0	8
Total cases	52	6	95	85	8	115
Frequency	5.8%	16.7%	15.8%	8.2%	0.0%	7.0%
Total minutes	366	83	1576	808	0	1278
Average additional minutes	7	14	17	10	0	11

$95 per patient of additional collections. Similarly, 7.0% to 8.2% of the Medicare total joints require additional surgery during the global period with $24 to $25, or an average $25 of additional collections (**Table 8**).

After discussions with the hospital, it is decided that the bundled payments will only apply to the commercial population. Based on the historical information of your practice, a bundled case rate for a 90-day global period is calculated by summing the average payment for the initial anesthesia procedures, additional services, and anesthesia for additional procedures as shown in **Table 9**. Your bundled payment price for all the services associated during that 90-day period at the current commercial payment level is $1525 per case.

Table 8
Anesthesia payments for additional surgical services in TJR 90-day global period

Additional Anesthesia Procedures Reported During Global Period	Commercial Payers ($)			Medicare ($)		
	Total Hip	Revised Total Hip	Total Knee	Total Hip	Revised Total Hip	Total Knee
00400 - Anesthesia for skin procedures	—	—	—	$188	—	—
01210 - Anesthesia for hip joint surgery	$648	—	—	$321	—	—
01214 - Anesthesia for hip arthroplasty	—	—	$1245	—	—	—
01215 - Anesthesia for revise hip repair	—	—	$1763	—	—	—
01220 - Anesthesia for Closed procedure on Femur	—	$1220	—	$280	—	—
01230 - Anesthesia for open surgery on femur	$708	—	$516	$350	—	—
01270 - Anesthesia for upper leg artery surgery	—	—	—	—	—	$581
01360 - Anesthesia for lower femur surgery	—	—	$896	—	—	$328
01380 - Anesthesia for knee joint closed procedure	—	—	$408	—	—	—
01392 - Anesthesia for knee area surgery	—	—	$411	—	—	—
01400 - Anesthesia for knee joint surgery	—	—	—	—	—	$204
01402 - Anesthesia for knee arthroplasty	$1148	—	$1148	—	—	$370
01480 - Anesthesia for lower leg surgery	$337	—	$631	$241	—	$241
Additional payments	$2504	$1220	$10,794	$2051	—	$2874
Additional procedures (n)	3	1	15	7	0	8
Average payment	$835	$1220	$720	$293	—	$359
Total TJR episodes (n)	52	6	95	85	8	115
Additional payment per TJR episode	$48	$203	$114	$24	—	$25

Abbreviation: TJR, total joint replacement.

Table 9
Average anesthesia payments per case for commercial patients in TJR 90-day global period

All Anesthesia Services Reported During 90-d TJR Episode	Cases (n)	Anesthesia for TJR Procedure Payment (See Table 4)	Additional CPT Services During TJR 90-d Period (See Table 6)	Additional Surgeries During TJR 90-d Period (See Table 8)	Total Payments During TJR 90-d Period
01214 - Anesthesia for hip arthroplasty	52	$1245	$113	$48	$1406
01215 - Anesthesia for revise hip repair	6	$1610	$190	$203	$2004
01402 - Anesthesia for knee arthroplasty	95	$1220	$227	$114	$1561
Average payment	153	$1244	$187	$95	$1525

Abbreviation: TJR, total joint replacement.

You have tracked the time associated with each of the activities: initial anesthesia for the surgical procedure, additional time for invasive monitoring and nerve blocks, along with the additional time associated with additional anesthesia for procedures within the 90-day surgical period (**Table 10**). Using the methods discussed herein to determine cost for the additional CPT services and additional surgeries the average additional time needed is 20 minutes. The average total joint case will require 148 minutes of time. You recognize that there is additional time that each case requires: preoperative evaluation (20 minutes), time in the PACU (10 minutes), time for evaluating the recovery from anesthesia (10 minutes), and perhaps pain medicine management (5 minutes), yielding an additional 45 minutes per case that is not directly captured by your data. We add the average time for additional services and the average time required when anesthesia for additional procedures is required (see **Table 10**). Each case takes an average of 198 minutes to perform.

You assumed that the cost of anesthesiologist time was $5 per minute, yielding the cost of performing a bundled average anesthesia service of $990 per case. Because this calculation is based on averages, you may want to calculate a confidence interval. Our sample size was 156 patients, with mean time of 194 minutes and assuming a 30 minutes standard deviation, our 99% confidence interval is 198 ± 4.1 minutes. Our average cost is likely $970 to $1110 per case.

Your starting point in bundled payment negotiations for all anesthesia services in patients undergoing hip and knee joint replacement is based on your current expected payments of $1525 (see **Table 9**). We know that, in many commercial populations, insurers pay approximately 80% and patients are responsible for the remaining 20%. Depending on your population, the actual payment rates may vary. For our example, let's assume that you can expect to collect 90% of the negotiated payment of $1518 or $1373. Assuming the upper confidence limit cost estimate, this establishes the range of payment you can accept in the negotiations: $1110-$1373. Any dollars above $1110 will likely contribute to margin. Strictly looking at the commercial cases, you cannot afford to accept a payment of less than $1100 per case.

Table 10
Average time per case for commercial patients in 90-d global period

All Anesthesia Services Reported During 90-d TJR Episode	Cases	Average Preservice and Postservice Time for Anesthesia Services	Average Time for Anesthesia Procedure (min) (See Table 2)	Average Time for Additional CPT Services (min) (See Table 5)	Average Time for Additional Surgery (min) (See Table 7)	Average Total Time for All Services (min)
01214 - Anesthesia for hip arthroplasty	52	45	129	10	7	191
01215 - Anesthesia for revise hip repair	6	45	202	4	14	265
01402 - Anesthesia for knee arthroplasty	95	45	124	12	17	198
Average time (min)	153	45	129	11	13	198

Abbreviation: TJR, total joint replacement.

Finally, you must recognize that the commercial patients essentially subsidize the losses incurred under Medicare payment rates. If you accept reductions in payment for the commercial, you erode the contributions to margin that those commercial cases represent. We recommend that you review the bundled payment price over all payers before accepting a bundled payment rate.

ALTERNATIVE PAYMENT MODEL OPPORTUNITIES

As we move into this next era of health care delivery and payment under the programs created by the Medicare Access and CHIP Reauthorization Act of 2015, we can anticipate expansion beyond accountable care organizations. Anesthesia literature contains many studies that demonstrate how an anesthetic technique or preoperative preparation can influence the patient's morbidity, mortality and length of stay. The new models of care and payment may provide an opportunity to reward an anesthesia group for the services it provides for which it currently does not receive payment. The perioperative surgical home may become a key tool in these models.

In 2009, a large Canadian study stated that anesthesia consultations before major noncardiac surgery reduced the duration of stay by 0.35 days.[10] Although it may be controversial, if routine anesthesia consultations decrease joint replacement patient's duration of stay by the same amount, this value is quantifiable. The Agency for Healthcare Research and Quality Healthcare Cost and Utilization Project Core Data (2011) lists daily inpatient hospital costs of $3300 per day.[11] A decrease of 0.35 days would decrease the direct hospital costs by $1155. In an accountable care organization model, this savings could be shared between the hospital and the anesthesiologists.

If this service were provided, there would also be an additional cost associated with setting up the anesthesia consultations. This is where a careful analysis of the costs of adding this service would have to be realized.

Anesthesiologists also influence patient outcomes and reduce durations of stay through pain management techniques, leading to early ambulation and fewer thromboembolic events, and intraoperative hypotensive techniques reducing blood loss and decreasing the need for costly blood products.

SUMMARY

It is possible for anesthesia practices to use their historical data and build a bundled payment based on some basic economic models. In this article, we used arithmetic means to estimate our payments, additional services, and additional surgical procedures. Although useful, groups should use more robust methods of approximation and include the statistical distribution of these events in their analysis.

The final estimate for a bundled payment of $1525 was more than 30% higher than the initial $1180 estimate based on an incomplete selection of joint replacement procedures and just the singular anesthetic procedure. When calculating bundled payments, groups need to account for all of the associated anesthetic services they provide in the entire global period, as well as the costs in delivering their service.

There are significant opportunities to apply our clinical expertise across the surgical episode of care. For too long, our contributions have been made without sufficient recognition. We need to leverage the tremendous research investment made by anesthesiologists, apply them to clinical care, and monetize the improvement in patient care. This practice becomes even more important under the payment systems put in place via the Medicare Access and CHIP Reauthorization Act. Medicare Access and CHIP Reauthorization Act's Quality Payment Program with its Merit-based Incentive Payment System and Alternative Payment Models includes an emphasis on both the costs and the quality of care and both of these will factor into payment calculations.

REFERENCES

1. Futurescan 2010: Healthcare trends and implications 2010-2015, Society for Healthcare Strategy and Market Development and the American College of Healthcare Executives with support from Thomson Reuters and VHA, Inc Health Administration Press; 2009.
2. American Society of Anesthesiologists (ASA). 2018 Relative Value Guide. Chicago (IL): American Society of Anesthesiologists, Inc; 2017.
3. Abouleish A, Stead SW, Cohen NA. Myth or fact: nurse anesthetists cost less than anesthesiologists. ASA Newsl 2010;74(12):30–4.
4. Centers for Medicare & Medicaid Services (CMS). Medicare fee-for-service payment. Available at: https://www.cms.gov/Medicare/Medicare-Fee-for-Service-Payment/PhysicianFeeSched/Downloads/2018-Anesthesia-Conversion-Factors.zip. Accessed November 12, 2017.
5. Kaplan RS, Anderson SR. Time-driven activity-based costing. Harv Bus Rev 2004;82(11):131–8.
6. Kaplan RS, Witkowski M, Abbott M, et al. Using time-driven activity-based costing to identify value improvement opportunities in healthcare. J Healthc Manag 2014;59(6):399–412.
7. DiGiola AM, Greenouse PK, Giarrusso ML, et al. Determining the true cost to deliver total hip and knee arthroplasty over the full cycle of care: preparing for bundling and reference-based pricing. J Arthroplasty 2016;31(1):1–6.
8. United States Government Accountability Office (GAO). Report GAO-07–463. Medicare physician payments – Medicare and private payment differences for anesthesia services. Available at: http://www.gao.gov/new.items/d07463.pdf. Accessed November 11, 2017.
9. Stead SW, Merrick SK. ASA survey results for commercial fees paid for anesthesia services - 2017. ASA Monitor 2017;81(10):64–71.
10. Wijeysundera DN, Austin PC, Beattie WS, et al. A population-based study of anesthesia consultation before major noncardiac surgery. Arch Intern Med 2009;169(6):595–602.
11. Weiss AJ, Elixhauser A, Andrews RM. Characteristics of operating room procedures in U.S. hospitals, 2011. HCUP statistical brief #170. Rockville (MD): Agency for Healthcare Research and Quality; 2014. Available at: http://www.hcup-us.ahrq.gov/reports/statbriefs/sb170-Operating-Room-Procedures-United-States-2011.pdf.

Comprehensive Preoperative Assessment and Global Optimization

Neil N. Shah, MD[a], Thomas R. Vetter, MD, MPH[b,c],*

KEYWORDS

- Preoperative assessment • Preoperative optimization • Telemedicine • Telehealth
- Medical comorbidity • Prehabilitation • Value-based health care

KEY POINTS

- The scope of preoperative management must be expanded to deliver greater value-based health care and to contribute to sustained and meaningful perioperative population health management.
- Preoperative risk factor assessment and stratification are essential for undertaking preoperative medical optimization via targeted, preemptive therapeutic interventions.
- Increasing use of telemedicine and telehealth, including mobile technologies and connectivity, are key to making health care more accessible, more cost effective, and of greater value.
- There are many comorbid conditions that represent perioperative risk factors that should be fully assessed and optimized before an elective and time-sensitive surgical procedure.
- Prehabilitation with a holistic approach that, in addition to physical exercise, includes nutritional and psychosocial support seems to be more effective at promoting postoperative functional recovery.

INTRODUCTION

In the United States and other Western nations, there is an ongoing evolution away from volume-based and toward value-based health care payment models.[1–3] Delivering value-based health care requires effectively managing not only the long-term

Disclosures: The authors have no relationship with a commercial company that has a direct financial interest in the subject matter or materials discussed in this article or with a company making a competing product.
^a Department of Medicine, Dell Medical School, The University of Texas at Austin, Health Discovery Building, 1701 Trinity Street, Austin, TX 78712-1875, USA; ^b Department of Surgery and Perioperative Care, Dell Medical School, The University of Texas at Austin, Health Discovery Building, Room 6.812, 1701 Trinity Street, Austin, TX 78712-1875, USA; ^c Department of Population Health, Dell Medical School, The University of Texas at Austin, Health Discovery Building, Room 6.812, 1701 Trinity Street, Austin, TX 78712-1875, USA
* Corresponding author.
E-mail address: thomas.vetter@austin.utexas.edu

Anesthesiology Clin 36 (2018) 259–280
https://doi.org/10.1016/j.anclin.2018.01.006
1932-2275/18/© 2018 Elsevier Inc. All rights reserved.

but also the short-term health of patient populations, especially high-risk patents and during disproportionately costly acute care episodes.[4-6] Managing the short-term health of the surgical population begins in the preoperative phase of care.[7,8]

According to the 2012 American Society of Anesthesiologists (ASA) Practice Advisory for Preanesthesia Evaluation, an anesthesiologist is responsible for medically assessing and optimizing a surgical patient.[9] Per the ASA advisory this involves "(1) discovery or identification of a disease or disorder that may affect perioperative anesthetic care; (2) verification or assessment of an already known disease, disorder, medical or alternative therapy that may affect perioperative anesthetic care; and (3) formulation of specific plans and alternatives for perioperative anesthetic care."[9]

However, to successfully deliver greater value-based care and to effectively contribute to sustained and meaningful perioperative population health management, the scope of existing preoperative management and its associated services and provider skills must be expanded.[7,8,10] This article focuses on the opportunities and mechanisms for delivering value-based, comprehensive preoperative assessment and global optimization of the surgical patient.

PREOPERATIVE RISK FACTOR ASSESSMENT AND STRATIFICATION

Preoperative risk factor assessment and stratification[11] is essential for undertaking preoperative medical optimization via targeted, preemptive therapeutic interventions. There are several global risk stratification tools available for major noncardiac surgery (eg, the Portsmouth-Physiology and Operative Severity Score for the enUmeration of Mortality and the Surgical Risk Scale).[11] However, despite its inherent subjectivity and only moderate interrater reliability in clinical practice,[12] the ASA physical status (PS) score continues to be conventionally used for overall preoperative risk assessment and stratification.

There are also numerous condition-specific risk screening and stratification tools applicable for patients undergoing noncardiac surgery (**Table 1**). Clinicians must prioritize which of these condition-specific tools to apply to avoid excessive patient respondent burden. Ideally, a condition-specific risk screening and stratification tool can be administered by telephone interview or self-completed via an online patient portal.

Stonemetz and Thomsen[13] at the Johns Hopkins Health System have innovated and successively revised their Preoperative Roadmap, which contains a Patient Evaluation Screening Form. Based on institutional clinician survey data and a consensus decision-making approach, Vetter and colleagues[14] at the University of Alabama at Birmingham generated a similar but more extensive Preoperative Patient Clearance and Consultation Screening Questionnaire.

In their prescient 2009 article on integrated preoperative assessment and consultation, Silverman and Rosenbaum[15] recommended the use of an integrated clinical risk profile matrix. Their 2-dimensional matrix included a uniform grading of existing patient morbidities versus the anticipated surgical disturbance (ie, surgical insult or surgical trespass).[15] Of note, the 2012 ASA Practice Advisory for Preanesthesia Evaluation also recommended stratifying patients on the level of surgical invasiveness (high, medium, or low) and the severity of disease (high or low).[9]

Vetter and colleagues[16] at the Dell Medical School and the Seton Healthcare Family have created an analogous Preoperative Patient Categorization and Management Matrix (**Fig. 1**), which incorporates (a) the number and significance of positive "red flags" on a locally revised version of the original University of Alabama at Birmingham Preoperative Patient Clearance and Consultation Screening Questionnaire[14] (**Fig. 2**) and

Table 1
Condition-specific risk screening and stratification tools that are applicable for patients undergoing noncardiac surgery

Tool	Condition
Lee Revised Cardiac Risk Index[110–112]	Cardiac complications
Gupta Cardiac Risk Calculator[113]	Myocardial infarction or cardiac arrest
University of California "3 Bucket" Model[114–116]	Deep venous thrombosis and venous thromboembolism
Rothman/Thomas Jefferson Joint Arthroplasty Risk Calculator[117]	Deep venous thrombosis and venous thromboembolism
STOP-Bang Questionnaire[118,119]	Obstructive sleep apnea
Patient Health Questionnaire (PHQ-2, PHQ-8, and PHQ-9)[120,121]	Depression
Generalized Anxiety Disorder Scale (GAD-2, GAD-7)[120,122,123]	Anxiety disorders
Mini-Cog[124,125]	Dementia (directly) and postoperative delirium (proxy)
Brief Screen for Cognitive Impairment (BSCI)[126–128]	Dementia (directly) and postoperative delirium (proxy)
Reported Edmonton Frail Scale (REFS)[129]	Frailty
Home Calculator[130]	Discharge disposition after surgery
Risk Assessment and Prediction Tool (RAPT)[131,132]	Discharge disposition after total joint arthroplasty
CAGE Questionnaire[133–135]	Alcohol use disorder
Alcohol Use Disorders Identification Test Consumption (AUDIT-C)[135,136]	Alcohol use disorder
Opioid Risk Tool (ORT)[137,138]	Opioid substance abuse and addiction
Screener and Opioid Assessment for Patients with Pain – Revised (SOAPP-R)[137,139,140]	Opioid substance abuse and addiction
Eight-Item Brief Form of the SOAPP-R (SOAPP-8)[141,142]	Opioid substance abuse and addiction

Comorbidity Based "Red Flags" on Preoperative Screening Questionnaire, Condition-Specific Screening Tools and/or ASA Physical Status Score ↓	Surgical Procedure Intensity Class 1 (1 = Minimal)	Surgical Procedure Intensity Class 2	Surgical Procedure Intensity Class 3	Surgical Procedure Intensity Class 4	Surgical Procedure Intensity Class 5 (5 = High)
1	EXPRESS	EXPRESS	EXPRESS	EXPRESS	EXPRESS
2	EXPRESS	EXPRESS	PASS	PASS	PASS
3	PASS	GO	GO	GO	GO
4	PASS	GO	GO	GO	GO

Fig. 1. Preoperative patient categorization and management matrix. ASA, American Society of Anesthesiologists. (*Courtesy of* T.R. Vetter, MD, MPH, Austin, TX.)

**Patient Preoperative Consultation
and Clearance Questionnaire**

Patient Information

Patient Name: _____   **Today's Date:** _____

Patient Date of Birth: _____   **Surgeon:** _____

In order to provide the very best care for you during your surgical experience at Seton, we ask that you answer the following questions about your medical conditions. Certain conditions may need special care for you, or change the timing of your surgery. It is very important to your care that you please answer these questions carefully and as accurately as possible. There is no right or wrong answer. Your answers are confidential (private). If you need help with this questionnaire, feel free to ask clinic staff or allow a family member to assist you. Thank you.

Do you currently have or ever had any of the following?		
HEART OR BLOOD VESSEL DISEASE	YES	NO
1. Too much fluid in your lungs (congestive heart failure)		
2. Heart attack (myocardial infarction)		
3. If you have had a heart attack, was it in the past 6 mo?		
4. Chest pain		
5. Shortness of breath		
6. Irregular, slow, or fast heart beat		
7. Heart murmur or heart valve problem (aortic stenosis, aortic regurgitation, mitral regurgitation, mitral valve prolapse, etc.)		
8. Any implanted devices in your heart (cardiac stents, heart valves, pacemaker or defibrillator)		
9. Heart or blood vessel surgery (coronary artery bypass, heart valve replacement or carotid artery surgery)		
10. High blood pressure in the lungs (pulmonary hypertension)		
11. Blood clots in legs or lungs (deep vein thrombosis, pulmonary embolus)		
12. Blood pressure reading greater than 160/100 (160 over 100) in past 6 mo		
13. Are you taking any blood thinner now? Examples include aspirin, Coumadin (warfarin), Plavix (clopidogrel), Effient (prasugrel), Pradaxa (dabigatran), Xarelto (rivaroxaban), Eliquis (apixaban)		
14. Have you seen a heart doctor (cardiologist) within the last y? If "YES," please provide the full name, address, and telephone number of your cardiologist: _____		
15. Are you unable to walk up 2 full flights of stairs or walk 4–6 city blocks *without stopping*? (Do not answer "YES" if the only reason that you are unable to do this is because of an orthopedic condition)		

Fig. 2. Preoperative patient clearance and consultation screening questionnaire. (*Courtesy of* T.R. Vetter, MD, MPH, Austin, TX.)

a subset of condition-specific risk screening tools (see **Table 1**) and (b) the intensity of the planned surgical procedure.

DESCRIPTION OF A PERIOPERATIVE ASSESSMENT AND GLOBAL OPTIMIZATION PROGRAM

Comprehensive perioperative management (eg, within a perioperative surgical home model) encompasses and seamlessly integrates the preoperative, intraoperative, postoperative, and postdischarge phases of care.[8,17,18] The goals are to optimize

Do you currently have or ever had any of the following?		
LUNG DISEASE	**YES**	**NO**
16. Chronic obstructive pulmonary disease (COPD), pulmonary fibrosis, cystic fibrosis, or frequent or severe asthma attacks		
17. Obstructive sleep apnea (OSA)		
18. Pneumonia in the past month (past 30 d)		
19. Do you use oxygen during the day or during the night?		
KIDNEY DISEASE	**YES**	**NO**
20. Chronic kidney disease		
21. Receive dialysis for your chronic kidney disease		
LIVER DISEASE	**YES**	**NO**
22. Chronic hepatitis, cirrhosis, or liver failure		
NERVOUS SYSTEM DISORDERS	**YES**	**NO**
23. Stroke, transient ischemic attack (TIA), brain aneurysm, Alzheimer's or dementia, Parkinson's, seizures, multiple sclerosis, or brain tumor		
JOINT OR MUSCLE DISORDERS	**YES**	**NO**
24. Rheumatoid arthritis (inflammatory arthritis)		
25. Myasthenia gravis or muscular dystrophy		
BLEEDING OR BLOOD DISORDERS	**YES**	**NO**
26. Hemophilia, von Willebrand disease, Factor II, V, VII, X, or XII deficiency		
27. Iron deficiency anemia		
28. Sickle cell anemia or thalassemia		
29. Do you bruise easily when bumped or bleed easily when cut or scraped		
ORGAN TRANSPLANT	**YES**	**NO**
30. Have you had an organ transplant?		
ALCOHOL OR STREET DRUGS	**YES**	**NO**
31. Do you drink alcohol heavily, meaning 5 or more drinks on the same occasion on 5 or more days in the past month (past 30 days)?		
32. Do you ever take narcotic prescription medications not prescribed for you?		
33. Do you ever use street (illicit) drugs?		
PREGNANCY	**YES**	**NO**
34. Are you pregnant or do you think you could be pregnant?		
CHRONIC PAIN	**YES**	**NO**
35. Do you take an opioid like Lortab/Norco/Vicodin or Percocet daily?		
36. Do you take a long-acting opioid like OxyContin, MS CONTIN, methadone, or Suboxone (buprenorphine)?		
ADVANCED AGE	**YES**	**NO**
37. Are you 80 y of age or older?		
ANESTHESIA PROBLEMS	**YES**	**NO**
38. Have you had any problems with having anesthesia in the past? For example: Was it hard for them to get the breathing tube in place? Was it hard for you to wake up? Did you have an allergic reaction to an anesthesia drug? Did you have a high fever because of the anesthesia drugs (malignant hyperthermia)?		
39. Have any of your close family members had an allergic reaction to an anesthesia drugs or had a high fever because of the anesthesia drugs (malignant hyperthermia)?		

Fig. 2. (*continued*).

not only surgical outcomes (quality and safety), but also the patient and provider experience.[8,16–18]

Our prototypic Perioperative Assessment and Global Optimization (PASS-GO) program is a central component of our institutional perioperative population health management.[16] Once the patient and the surgeon decide to pursue surgery, the PASS-GO process is initiated.

All surgical patients undergo an initial, brief pre-admission testing visit for routine vital signs (including height, weight, neck circumference, and oxygen saturation in room air); standardized, evidence-based laboratory testing, electrocardiogram, and nasal swab culture; and, if desired, an in-person patient education class. All patients are then interviewed via telephone by a specially trained registered nurse in our fully integrated Perioperative Command Center. This collected information is entered into an individualized preoperative dashboard in the patient's electronic medical record and, thus, made available to the surgeon, anesthesiologist, hospitalist, primary care physician, and all other care providers.[16]

Based on the data collected via the preadmission testing visit and initial telephone patient interview, the patient is stratified by an advanced practice registered nurse or physician assistant, also located in our centralized Perioperative Command Center, into 1 of 3 categories or "swim lanes" that are referred to as EXPRESS, PASS, or GO (see **Fig. 1**; **Fig. 3**). As needed, this advanced practice provider confers with a designated anesthesiologist and/or internal medicine hospitalist—who function equally as the perioperativist. Postdischarge disposition and a postacute care plan are also initially determined with the patient and any available, designated domestic "copilot." This process can entail a home site visit by a Perioperative Command Center social worker and/or health promoter.[16]

This patient categorization (EXPRESS, PASS, or GO) is determined by the combination of (a) significant preoperative comorbidities or risk factors, which are identified on the preoperative clearance and consult questionnaire (see **Fig. 2**), along with the results of a subset of preoperative screening tools (see **Table 1**) and (b) the expected level of surgical intensity, based on its invasiveness, physiologic stress, estimated blood loss, and a planned postoperative intensive care unit admission.[9,13–16]

Patients with no or minimal comorbidities or risk factors (ASA PS 1) are deemed eligible for EXPRESS status (see **Fig. 1**). EXPRESS patients can be immediately and definitively scheduled for their planned surgery, undergo an additional brief telephone

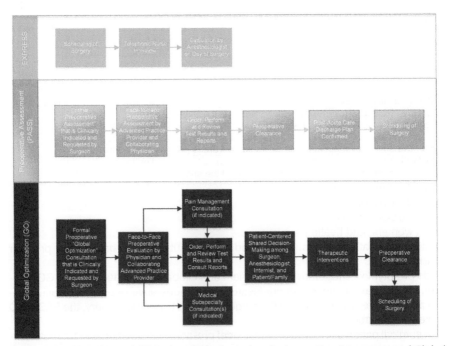

Fig. 3. EXPRESS, PASS, and GO Patient Swim Lanes in a Perioperative Assessment and Global Optimization (PASS-GO) program. (*Courtesy of* T.R. Vetter, MD, MPH, Austin, TX.)

interview with an anesthesia care team nurse, and are evaluated on the day of surgery by an anesthesiologist (see **Fig. 3**).[16]

Patients with moderate comorbid risk factors (ASA PS 2 or 3) are categorized as needing preoperative assessment (PASS; see **Fig. 1**). PASS patients have a face-to-face, preoperative evaluation and management encounter with an advanced practice provider, collaborating closely with a designated perioperativist (anesthesiologist or hospitalist). Based on the patient's specific needs, additional diagnostic tests are performed, and the results reviewed with the patient and surgeon. Once a PASS patient receives formal preoperative anesthesia clearance, the initially tentative scheduled surgery date and postacute care discharge plan are confirmed (see **Fig. 3**).[16]

Patients with major comorbid risk factors (ASA PS 3 or 4) are categorized as needing Global Optimization (GO) (see **Fig. 1**). GO patients have a face-to-face, preoperative evaluation and management consultation with an anesthesiologist or hospitalist (perioperativist). After this consultation, the patient may undergo advanced diagnostic testing, along with a pain management consultation and medical subspecialty consultations. The surgeon and other perioperative team members may engage with the patient and family in a shared decision-making process about possible alternative therapeutic options to surgery (eg, long-term medical management). The final decision whether to proceed with surgery is made (see **Fig. 3**). If the providers and patient/family mutually agree to proceed with surgery—and once the patient has undergone any necessary therapeutic interventions, has been medically optimized, and received formal preoperative anesthesia clearance—the surgery is definitively scheduled and the postacute care discharge plan is confirmed (see **Fig. 3**).[16]

ROLE OF TELEMEDICINE AND TELEHEALTH

With ongoing national health reform in the United States, millions more individuals are gaining access to a health care system that is concomitantly grappling to provide continued high-quality care at reduced costs.[19,20] Increasing the use of medical informatics as well as mobile technologies and connectivity are viewed as key strategies for making health care more accessible, more cost effective, and of greater value.[19,21] There has, thus, been a surge in interest in and use of telemedicine and telehealth, catalyzed by the continued expectations and rewards for greater efficiency in health care delivery.[20,22]

Enhanced preoperative assessment and optimization requires rigorous interdisciplinary support and collaboration outside a single setting and point in time.[23] Telemedicine and telehealth can facilitate this longitudinal, highly interactive, yet often ideally virtual care requirement.

In our own multifacility and geographically dispersed health care system, our Perioperative Command Center is pivotal to our PASS-GO Program. The nurse navigators, social workers, and health promoters in this Perioperative Command Center provide multiple telephonic patient touch-points across the entire perioperative continuum (**Fig. 4**). Patients are strongly encouraged to contact the Perioperative Command Center day or night with any questions or concerns before and especially after their surgery. This contact includes calling before they present to an emergency department and possibly are readmitted to an acute care hospital.

We have created an organizational hub-and-spoke perioperative care delivery system, in which an advanced practice provider and a surgical patient, who are physically located in a satellite PASS-GO clinic (the spoke), both interact virtually with an attending anesthesiologist or hospitalist (perioperativist) in our central PASS-GO clinic

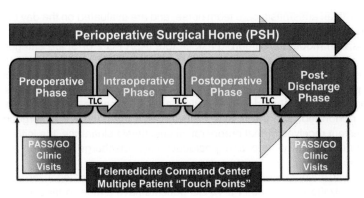

Fig. 4. Operationalizing a Perioperative Assessment and Global Optimization (PASS-GO) Program, including its transitions across levels of care (TLC) service and perioperative command center. (*Courtesy of* T.R. Vetter, MD, MPH, Austin, TX.)

(the hub). This real-time, high-fidelity audiovisual interaction includes the technology to remotely auscultate the patient's heart, lungs, and carotid arteries.

CONVENTIONAL COMORBID RISK FACTOR OPTIMIZATION

There are many comorbid conditions that represent perioperative risk factors that should be fully assessed and optimized before undergoing an elective and time-sensitive surgical procedure (**Box 1**). We have elected to focus here on a representative subset, but especially burgeoning prehabilitation.

The definitions of an urgent versus time-sensitive versus elective procedure are often debated among providers. The 2014 American College of Cardiology/American Heart Association Guideline on Perioperative Cardiovascular Evaluation and Management of Patients Undergoing Noncardiac Surgery[24] provides useful definitions and guidance in this regard (**Table 2**), thus, clarifying the windows of opportunity for preoperative assessment and optimization.

Coronary Artery Disease

Cardiovascular disease remains the leading cause of death in the United States and worldwide.[25–27] An estimated 15.5 million or 6.2% of Americans 20 years of age or older have coronary artery disease.[26,27] Not surprisingly, the incidence of perioperative myocardial infarction (PMI) complicating noncardiac surgery ranges from 5% to 16% in more recent series; however, this event rate has not changed significantly over the last 2 decades.[28] PMI at the time of noncardiac surgery is associated with substantial mortality, morbidity, and additional health care costs.[29,30]

PMI results from acute inflammatory, hypercoagulable, hypoxic, and stress states.[29,30] Specifically, PMI occurs from either reduced coronary blood flow owing to an acute coronary artery plaque rupture and thrombosis (type 1) or a primary increase in oxygen demand in the setting of stable but fixed, stenotic coronary artery lesion(s) (type 2).[28] PMI results not only from "demand ischemia," but also in an estimated nearly 60% of cases from acute plaque rupture.[28]

It is also well-recognized that many surgical patients experience "silent" perioperative myocardial ischemia or infarction without any overt signs or symptoms.[29,31,32] A growing body of data supports the closely related phenomenon of and major mortality associated with myocardial injury after noncardiac surgery, detected only by a postoperative elevation in serum high-sensitivity troponin T.[33–38]

Box 1
Comorbid conditions that represent perioperative risk factors that should be fully assessed and optimized before undergoing an elective and time-sensitive surgical procedure

Coronary artery disease

Cardiomyopathy

Congestive heart failure

Arterial hypertension

Pulmonary hypertension

Cerebrovascular disease

Obstructive sleep apnea

Chronic obstructive pulmonary disease

Tobacco use

Diabetes and glycemic control

Overweight and obesity

Chronic liver disease

Chronic kidney disease

Anemia

Frailty

Cognitive dysfunction and dementia

Opioid use, misuse and abuse

However, current guidelines provide few recommendations on how to preoperatively to identify and manage patients who are at risk and/or demonstrate myocardial injury after noncardiac surgery.[38] Therefore, perioperative clinicians are currently limited to appreciating the importance of myocardial injury after noncardiac surgery

---

Table 2
Description of the temporal necessity of surgical procedures and windows of opportunity for preoperative assessment and optimization

Type of Procedure	Definition
Emergency procedure	"One in which life or limb is threatened if not in the operating room where there is time for no or very limited or minimal clinical evaluation, typically within <6 h."
Urgent procedure	"One in which there may be time for a limited clinical evaluation, usually when life or limb is threatened if not in the operating room, typically between 6 and 24 h."
Time-sensitive procedure	"One in which a delay of >1–6 wk to allow for an evaluation and significant changes in management will negatively affect outcome. Most oncologic procedures would fall into this category."
Elective procedure	"One in which the procedure could be delayed for up to 1 y."

Data from Fleisher LA, Fleischmann KE, Auerbach AD, et al. 2014 ACC/AHA guideline on perioperative cardiovascular evaluation and management of patients undergoing noncardiac surgery: a report of the American College of Cardiology/American Heart Association Task Force on Practice Guidelines. Circulation 2014;130(24):e278–333.

and applying recommendations based on observational data or derived from the nonoperative setting.[39]

Because the majority of noncardiac surgeries are elective, an accurate estimation of the risk of a perioperative cardiac event is important to allow informed patient and physician decision making.[24,29] Furthermore, major emphasis should be placed on prevention of and surveillance for major perioperative ischemic cardiac events in patients undergoing noncardiac surgery.[24,29,30] Much of these efforts are under the purview of comprehensive preoperative assessment and global optimization.

Anemia

Preoperative anemia is a common condition among surgical patients. However, its reported prevalence varies widely, ranging from 5% to 75%, depending on the type of surgery, the patient's age, gender, and comorbidities, as well as the criteria used for defining anemia.[40,41]

Preoperative anemia is independently associated with worse clinical outcomes in noncardiac surgery patients.[41–44] Published data also support a major independent association between intraoperative allogeneic blood transfusion and increased 30-day and longer term morbidity and mortality in patients undergoing noncardiac surgery.[45,46]

Comprehensive preoperative assessment and optimization provides an opportunity for proactive recognition and management of the anemia, thus, promoting patient blood management by mitigating the need for allogeneic blood transfusion and the risk of symptomatic postoperative anemia.[41,47–49]

Anemia screening should occur at least 30 days before the planned surgery so that appropriate anemia management can be initiated.[40,49–51] Anemia screening should be individualized based on a patient's symptoms, age, and comorbidities, type of surgery, and anticipated blood loss.[41]

Preoperative anemia should be viewed as a serious and treatable medical condition, rather than simply an abnormal laboratory value.[50,52] Therefore, the diagnosis of unexplained anemia in patients scheduled for elective surgery in which significant blood loss is anticipated should be considered an indication for rescheduling surgery until further differential diagnostic testing and appropriate nontransfusion treatment are completed.[49,50,53] Specifically, treatment of iron-deficiency anemia can include cost-effective, sequential preoperative doses of an erythropoiesis-stimulating agent (eg, epoetin alfa) and intravenous iron preparation (eg, iron sucrose).[54–56]

Diabetes and Glycemic Control

Diabetes has an estimated prevalence of 9.1% in adults in the United States[57] and is an independent risk factor for postoperative complications like surgical site infections and mortality.[58,59] The primary actionable benefit of identifying preoperative diabetes is reducing perioperative hyperglycemia,[60] which is associated with increased mortality, myocardial infarction, acute renal failure, infection, increased duration of stay, readmission, and overall hospital costs.[61–63] The level of hyperglycemia directly correlates with risk,[61] and effective control with insulin reduces risk in a dose-dependent relationship.[63] Although identifying preoperative diabetes is beneficial, up to 30% of perioperative hyperglycemia occurs in patients without diabetes[63] and is associated with an even greater increased risk.[64]

Elevated preoperative hemoglobin A1C levels are associated with poor perioperative glycemic control.[60] Although routine testing of patients is not recommended,[59] risk factors such as age greater than 45 years or a body mass index of greater than 25 kg/m^2 can guide diabetes screening.[65] Patients undergoing vascular and orthopedic surgery are at increased risk of cardiac events and infectious complications, thus likely warranting hemoglobin A1C screening for undiagnosed diabetes.[59] Patients with known diabetes should have their hemoglobin A1C level measured once during the 3 months preceding surgery to determine the level of glycemic control and associated risk. Identifying nondiabetic patients at risk of perioperative hyperglycemia is more challenging, but risk factors in cardiac surgery patients include advanced age, male gender, obesity, preoperative creatinine, history of prior cardiac surgery, reduced ejection fraction, and cardiogenic shock.[66]

Although the adverse effects of preoperative diabetes and perioperative hyperglycemia are clear, data-driven management recommendations are sparse. If time permits, improving long-term diabetic control before surgery is reasonable, because diabetics with preoperative hemoglobin A1C values between 6.5% and 8.0% have a decreased duration of stay.[67] However, there is insufficient evidence to postpone surgery for uncontrolled diabetes unless there is concern for diabetic ketoacidosis or hyperosmolar nonketotic state, which are medical emergencies.[65]

Oral hypoglycemic agents should be held on the day of surgery, and long-acting insulin should be dose reduced by 20% to 50%.[68] Blood glucose should be checked on the day of surgery with a target range for most patients between 80 and 180 mg/dL.[65] Patients with levels above this threshold should be treated with short-acting insulin and undergo glucose monitoring every 4 to 6 hours.[68] Critically ill patients may benefit from intensive glycemic control with an insulin infusion protocol set to target blood glucose between 100 and 150 mg/dL.[69,70]

Opioid Use, Misuse, and Abuse

Logically within the framework of the perioperative surgical home,[71–73] anesthesiologists and other pain medicine specialists are well-qualified and uniquely positioned to develop, implement, and coordinate a comprehensive perioperative analgesic plan, which begins with formal preoperative patient assessment and optimization and continues throughout the postdischarge, convalescence period.[73] However, the scope of perioperative pain management practice needs to:

a. Expand to include routine preoperative patient-level pain risk stratification, including the chronic use, misuse, or abuse of opioid and nonopioid analgesics;
b. Address the multitude of biopsychosocial factors that contribute to interpatient pain variability; and
c. Extend and be well-coordinated across all 4 (preoperative, intraoperative, postoperative and postdischarge) phases of the surgical pain experience.[71–75]

Specifically, safe and effective perioperative pain management should include a plan of care that is tailored to the individual patient's underlying disease(s); presence of a chronic pain condition; the preoperative use, misuse or abuse of opioids; and the specific surgical procedure—with an evidence-based, opioid-sparing, multimodal analgesic regimen being applied in the vast majority of cases.[71–73,76–78]

PREHABILITATION

Prehabilitation is the process of enhancing functional capacity before undergoing a physical stressor and is a growing area of preoperative optimization.[79] Instead of focusing only on postoperative rehabilitative recovery, prehabilitation capitalizes on the preoperative period to strengthen patients and to mitigate postoperative functional decline. Compared with rehabilitation alone, the addition of prehabilitation can significantly increase postoperative functional capacity.[80]

Frailty is defined as a decreased physiologic reserve, leading to an increased vulnerability to stressors like surgery, and is a growing concern as more elderly patients undergo surgery.[81] Although there is no universally accepted method of quantifying preoperative frailty, the Edmonton Frail Scale or Reported Edmonton Frail Scale seems to be able to risk stratify and highlight aspects of frailty that are amenable to preoperative optimization.[81] Frailty as an independent risk factor for adverse perioperative outcomes is becoming quite apparent—further emphasizing the key role of prehabilitation.[81–83]

Prehabilitation has been shown to improve value-based health care outcomes like postoperative complications, hospital duration of stay, and patient satisfaction.[84–86] Published systematic reviews and meta-analyses on prehabilitation support improvements in postoperative physical function.[87–90] Furthermore, a cost-effectiveness analysis of an integrated prehabilitation/rehabilitation program showed a 15% overall cost reduction, despite the higher upfront expense owing to a shorter duration of hospital stay, decreased postoperative care use, and faster return to work.[91]

Whereas early prehabilitation programs focused primarily on physical exercise, a holistic approach including nutritional and psychosocial support seems to be more effective at promoting postoperative functional recovery than exercise alone.[92] Multimodal prehabilitation programs can improve postoperative functional capacity,[80,93] including one in which 81% of patients returned to baseline functional capacity 8 weeks after surgery versus only 40% of control subjects.[94]

Physical Exercise

Regular strenuous activity over time builds physiologic reserve and prepares the body to better handle the stress of surgery.[79] Early prehabilitation programs focused on physical exercise, which is particularly important in frail and elderly surgical patients.[82,89] Patients with poor baseline functional status can be identified with a 6-minute walking test distance of less than 400 m and are more likely to improve with prehabilitation programs.[95] Physiologic measurements like cardiopulmonary exercise testing, which measures expired gas and ventilatory flow during activity, can also be used to predict poor outcomes and guide exercise-based interventions.[96,97]

Prehabilitation exercise protocols vary but a reasonable program consists of 75 to 150 minutes of moderate to vigorous exercise per week, ideally divided into short frequent sessions. Exercise intensity can be measured subjectively with measures like the Borg Scale, which rates perceived exertion from 0 to 10.[79] Simple protocols, such as walking and breathing exercise programs, may be preferable to complex protocols owing to improved adherence.[98] General cardiopulmonary conditioning is likely beneficial for all major surgery, but exercise interventions should be tied to the specific planned procedure. For example, thoracic surgery should include a focus on aerobic and breathing exercise, whereas orthopedic surgery should include muscle strengthening.[79]

Nutritional Support

Surgery induces a stress state of catabolism with increased nutritional requirements and can lead to sarcopenia.[99] Additionally, many patients are already malnourished before surgery owing to their underlying medical condition(s). Preoperative malnutrition is associated with increased postoperative risk of unplanned admissions to the intensive care unit, prolonged intubation, acute renal failure, blood transfusion, infection, increased duration of stay, readmissions, and mortality.[100–103] Perioperative nutritional management can optimize preoperative nutritional status and provide protection against the impending catabolic stress of surgery. Nutritional therapy also improves exercise capacity, thereby enhancing the effect of exercise interventions.[79,102]

Although nutritional support can mitigate the catabolic effect of any major surgery, it should be guided by patient characteristics, medical condition, and type of procedure, especially when protein absorption and metabolism are involved.[102] For example, elderly patients with cancer undergoing abdominal surgery have a particularly high malnutrition risk.[104] The European Society for Clinical Nutrition and Metabolism surgical guidelines define patients at severe surgical risk with either:

a. Weight loss greater than 10% to 15% within 6 months,
b. Body mass index of less than 18.5 kg/m^2,
c. Serum albumin of less than 3 g/dL (without evidence of renal or hepatic dysfunction), or
d. Subjective Global Assessment grade of C or Nutritional Risk Screening score of greater than 5.[105]

Frailty indicators may also help to identify patients who would benefit from nutritional support.[82]

Patients with nutritional risk can benefit from dietician consultation and should begin oral protein and carbohydrate nutritional supplementation as soon as this is identified, but ideally at least 7 to 14 days before surgery.[99,102] The European Society for Clinical Nutrition and Metabolism guidelines also recommend avoiding long periods of preoperative fasting.[105] Although still widely practiced, fasting after midnight before surgery is no longer recommended. Clear carbohydrate drinks can be safely consumed up to 2 hours before surgery and can decrease the insulin resistance related to surgical stress, and increase patient comfort.[102]

Psychological Support

Surgery and the underlying illness may also cause significant emotional stress that can affect the need for hospitalization, duration of stay, infection, and wound healing.[79] Patients with preexisting psychiatric illness are likely at greater increased risk and should assuredly be optimized preoperatively.

Interventions include stress/anxiety management techniques like positive visualization, or relaxation/breathing exercises taught by a psychologist.[80,94,106] Psychological support can enhance adherence to exercise and nutrition recommendations.[107] Likewise, physical exercise itself can reduce psychological stress as a secondary benefit, supporting a multimodal approach.[79]

Practical Considerations

Using many of the methods described herein, patients at high risk for postoperative functional decline can be identified in the preoperative period and an appropriate prehabilitation program can be implemented. Although the optimal duration of a prehabilitation program has not been established, most studied protocols range between 4 and 8 weeks, with the timeline predicated by the chronicity of the underlying medical condition.[79,108] Adherence is a major factor in the success of any program and should be considered when designing the program timeline.[98] Ultimately, this planning may be predicated on the need for timely surgical intervention (see **Table 2**).

SUMMARY

The combined effects of expanded health insurance coverage, continued economic growth, and an aging population (the "silver tsunami") are expected to result in greater demand for health care goods and services in the United States by 2023 and almost certainly beyond.[17,109] This demand will include an increased need for and volume of surgical and perioperative care. There will be concomitant demands from stakeholders for a maximum return on investment—greater realized "value"—for this surgical and perioperative care. Comprehensive preoperative assessment and global optimization will play a pivotal role in delivering this higher quality and lower cost care to surgical patients.

REFERENCES

1. Thaker NG, Feeley TW. Creating the healthcare transformation from volume to value. In: Phillips RA, editor. America's healthcare transformation: strategies and innovations. New Brunswick (NJ): Rutgers University Press; 2016. p. 295–318.
2. Gordon JE, Leiman JM, Deland EL, et al. Delivering value: provider efforts to improve the quality and reduce the cost of health care. Annu Rev Med 2014; 65:447–58.
3. Stadhouders N, Koolman X, Tanke M, et al. Policy options to contain healthcare costs: a review and classification. Health Policy 2016;120(5):486–94.
4. Peterson TA, Bernstein SJ, Spahlinger DA. Population health: a new paradigm for medicine. Am J Med Sci 2016;351(1):26–32.
5. Steenkamer BM, Drewes HW, Heijink R, et al. Defining population health management: a scoping review of the literature. Popul Health Manag 2017;20(1):74–85.
6. Andrieni JD. Population health management: the lynchpin of emerging healthcare delivery models. In: Phillips RA, editor. America's healthcare transformation: strategies and innovations. New Brunswick (NJ): Rutgers University Press; 2016. p. 113–27.
7. Boudreaux AM, Vetter TR. A primer on population health management and its perioperative application. Anesth Analg 2016;123(1):63–70.
8. Vetter TR, Boudreaux AM, Jones KA, et al. The perioperative surgical home: how anesthesiology can collaboratively achieve and leverage the triple aim in health care. Anesth Analg 2014;118(5):1131–6.
9. Apfelbaum JL, Connis RT, Nickinovich DG, et al. Practice advisory for preanesthesia evaluation: an updated report by the American Society of Anesthesiologists Task Force on Preanesthesia Evaluation. Anesthesiology 2012;116(3): 522–38.
10. Alem N, Kain Z. Evolving healthcare delivery paradigms and the optimization of 'value' in anesthesiology. Curr Opin Anaesthesiol 2017;30(2):223–9.
11. Moonesinghe SR, Mythen MG, Das P, et al. Risk stratification tools for predicting morbidity and mortality in adult patients undergoing major surgery: qualitative systematic review. Anesthesiology 2013;119(4):959–81.
12. Sankar A, Johnson SR, Beattie WS, et al. Reliability of the American Society of Anesthesiologists physical status scale in clinical practice. Br J Anaesth 2014; 113(3):424–32.
13. Stonemetz J, Thomsen R. Preoperative roadmap: for providers requiring anesthesia services. 2016:1–17. Available at: http://anesthesiology.hopkinsmedicine.org/wp-content/uploads/2016/06/Preoperative-Roadmap-05_18_2016.pdf. Accessed October 17, 2017.
14. Vetter TR, Boudreaux AM, Ponce BA, et al. Development of a preoperative patient clearance and consultation screening questionnaire. Anesth Analg 2016; 123(6):1453–7.

15. Silverman DG, Rosenbaum SH. Integrated assessment and consultation for the preoperative patient. Med Clin North Am 2009;93(5):963–77.
16. Vetter TR, Uhler LM, Bozic KJ. Value-based healthcare: Preoperative Assessment and Global Optimization (PASS-GO): improving value in total joint replacement care. Clin Orthop Relat Res 2017;475(8):1958–62.
17. Vetter TR, Jones KA. Perioperative surgical home: perspective II. Anesthesiol Clin 2015;33(4):771–84.
18. Kain ZN, Vakharia S, Garson L, et al. The perioperative surgical home as a future perioperative practice model. Anesth Analg 2014;118(5):1126–30.
19. Kvedar J, Coye MJ, Everett W. Connected health: a review of technologies and strategies to improve patient care with telemedicine and telehealth. Health Aff (Millwood) 2014;33(2):194–9.
20. Gorevic J. Telemedicine: virtually redefining the delivery of care. In: Phillips RA, editor. America's healthcare transformation: strategies and innovations. New Brunswick (NJ): Rutgers University Press; 2016. p. 163–77.
21. Kim JY, Steinhubl SR. Medicine unplugged: can M-health transform. In: Phillips RA, editor. America's healthcare transformation: strategies and innovations. New Brunswick, NJ: Rutgers University Press; 2016. p. 142–62.
22. Weinstein RS, Lopez AM, Joseph BA, et al. Telemedicine, telehealth, and mobile health applications that work: opportunities and barriers. Am J Med 2014;127(3):183–7.
23. Brady JM. Evolving perioperative care team collaboration. J Perianesth Nurs 2017;32(5):490–3.
24. Fleisher LA, Fleischmann KE, Auerbach AD, et al. 2014 ACC/AHA guideline on perioperative cardiovascular evaluation and management of patients undergoing noncardiac surgery: a report of the American College of Cardiology/American Heart Association Task Force on Practice Guidelines. Circulation 2014;130(24):e278–333.
25. Santulli G. Epidemiology of cardiovascular disease in the 21st century: updated numbers and updated facts. J Cardiovasc Dis 2013;1(1):1–2.
26. Mozaffarian D, Benjamin EJ, Go AS, et al. Heart disease and stroke statistics-2016 update: a report from the American Heart Association. Circulation 2016;133(4):e38–360.
27. Mozaffarian D, Benjamin EJ, Go AS, et al. Executive summary: heart disease and stroke statistics–2016 update: a report from the American Heart Association. Circulation 2016;133(4):447–54.
28. Hanson I, Kahn J, Dixon S, et al. Angiographic and clinical characteristics of type 1 versus type 2 perioperative myocardial infarction. Catheter Cardiovasc Interv 2013;82(4):622–8.
29. Devereaux PJ, Goldman L, Cook DJ, et al. Perioperative cardiac events in patients undergoing noncardiac surgery: a review of the magnitude of the problem, the pathophysiology of the events and methods to estimate and communicate risk. CMAJ 2005;173(6):627–34.
30. Devereaux PJ, Sessler DI. Cardiac complications in patients undergoing major noncardiac surgery. N Engl J Med 2015;373(23):2258–69.
31. Devereaux PJ, Xavier D, Pogue J, et al. Characteristics and short-term prognosis of perioperative myocardial infarction in patients undergoing noncardiac surgery: a cohort study. Ann Intern Med 2011;154(8):523–8.
32. Sessler DI, Devereaux PJ. Perioperative troponin screening. Anesth Analg 2016;123(2):359–60.

33. van Waes JA, Nathoe HM, de Graaff JC, et al. Myocardial injury after noncardiac surgery and its association with short-term mortality. Circulation 2013;127(23): 2264–71.

34. Botto F, Alonso-Coello P, Chan MT, et al. Myocardial injury after noncardiac surgery: a large, international, prospective cohort study establishing diagnostic criteria, characteristics, predictors, and 30-day outcomes. Anesthesiology 2014;120(3):564–78.

35. Devereaux PJ, Biccard BM, Sigamani A, et al. Association of postoperative high-sensitivity troponin levels with myocardial injury and 30-day mortality among patients undergoing noncardiac surgery. JAMA 2017;317(16):1642–51.

36. Khan J, Alonso-Coello P, Devereaux PJ. Myocardial injury after noncardiac surgery. Curr Opin Cardiol 2014;29(4):307–11.

37. Devereaux PJ, Chan MT, Alonso-Coello P, et al. Association between postoperative troponin levels and 30-day mortality among patients undergoing noncardiac surgery. JAMA 2012;307(21):2295–304.

38. Horr S, Reed G, Menon V. Troponin elevation after noncardiac surgery: significance and management. Cleve Clin J Med 2015;82(9):595–602.

39. Mauermann E, Puelacher C, Lurati Buse G. Myocardial injury after noncardiac surgery: an underappreciated problem and current challenges. Curr Opin Anaesthesiol 2016;29(3):403–12.

40. Bisbe E, Muñoz M. Management of preoperative anemia: the NATA consensus statements. ISBT Sci Ser 2012;7(1):283–7.

41. Kansagra AJ, Stefan MS. Preoperative anemia: evaluation and treatment. Anesthesiol Clin 2016;34(1):127–41.

42. Baron DM, Hochrieser H, Posch M, et al. Preoperative anaemia is associated with poor clinical outcome in non-cardiac surgery patients. Br J Anaesth 2014;113(3):416–23.

43. Fowler AJ, Ahmad T, Phull MK, et al. Meta-analysis of the association between preoperative anaemia and mortality after surgery. Br J Surg 2015;102(11): 1314–24.

44. Musallam KM, Tamim HM, Richards T, et al. Preoperative anaemia and postoperative outcomes in non-cardiac surgery: a retrospective cohort study. Lancet 2011;378(9800):1396–407.

45. Glance LG, Dick AW, Mukamel DB, et al. Association between intraoperative blood transfusion and mortality and morbidity in patients undergoing noncardiac surgery. Anesthesiology 2011;114(2):283–92.

46. Smilowitz NR, Oberweis BS, Nukala S, et al. Association between anemia, bleeding, and transfusion with long-term mortality following noncardiac surgery. Am J Med 2016;129(3):315–23.e2.

47. Shander A, Bracey AW Jr, Goodnough LT, et al. Patient blood management as standard of care. Anesth Analg 2016;123(4):1051–3.

48. Meybohm P, Richards T, Isbister J, et al. Patient blood management bundles to facilitate implementation. Transfus Med Rev 2017;31(1):62–71.

49. Goodnough LT, Shander A. Patient blood management. Anesthesiology 2012; 116(6):1367–76.

50. Goodnough LT, Manaitis A, Earnshaw P, Nata Consensus Development Working Group. Management of preoperative anaemia in patients undergoing elective surgery. ISBT Sci Ser 2010;5(1):120–4.

51. Gombotz H. Patient blood management: a patient-orientated approach to blood replacement with the goal of reducing anemia, blood loss and the need for blood transfusion in elective surgery. Transfus Med Hemother 2012;39(2):67–72.

52. Goodnough LT, Maniatis A, Earnshaw P, et al. Detection, evaluation, and management of preoperative anaemia in the elective orthopaedic surgical patient: NATA guidelines. Br J Anaesth 2011;106(1):13–22.

53. Goodnough LT, Shander A, Spivak JL, et al. Detection, evaluation, and management of anemia in the elective surgical patient. Anesth Analg 2005;101(6):1858–61.

54. Lin DM, Lin ES, Tran MH. Efficacy and safety of erythropoietin and intravenous iron in perioperative blood management: a systematic review. Transfus Med Rev 2013;27(4):221–34.

55. Rineau E, Chaudet A, Chassier C, et al. Implementing a blood management protocol during the entire perioperative period allows a reduction in transfusion rate in major orthopedic surgery: a before-after study. Transfusion 2016;56(3):673–81.

56. Guinn NR, Guercio JR, Hopkins TJ, et al. How do we develop and implement a preoperative anemia clinic designed to improve perioperative outcomes and reduce cost? Transfusion 2016;56(2):297–303.

57. Myers CA, Slack T, Broyles ST, et al. Diabetes prevalence is associated with different community factors in the diabetes belt versus the rest of the United States. Obesity (Silver Spring) 2017;25(2):452–9.

58. Martin ET, Kaye KS, Knott C, et al. Diabetes and risk of surgical site infection: a systematic review and meta-analysis. Infect Control Hosp Epidemiol 2016;37(1):88–99.

59. Bock M, Johansson T, Fritsch G, et al. The impact of preoperative testing for blood glucose concentration and haemoglobin A1c on mortality, changes in management and complications in noncardiac elective surgery: a systematic review. Eur J Anaesthesiol 2015;32(3):152–9.

60. Perna M, Romagnuolo J, Morgan K, et al. Preoperative hemoglobin A1c and postoperative glucose control in outcomes after gastric bypass for obesity. Surg Obes Relat Dis 2012;8(6):685–90.

61. Frisch A, Chandra P, Smiley D, et al. Prevalence and clinical outcome of hyperglycemia in the perioperative period in noncardiac surgery. Diabetes Care 2010;33(8):1783–8.

62. Buehler L, Fayfman M, Alexopoulos AS, et al. The impact of hyperglycemia and obesity on hospitalization costs and clinical outcome in general surgery patients. J Diabetes Complications 2015;29(8):1177–82.

63. Kwon S, Thompson R, Dellinger P, et al. Importance of perioperative glycemic control in general surgery: a report from the surgical care and outcomes assessment program. Ann Surg 2013;257(1):8–14.

64. Kotagal M, Symons RG, Hirsch IB, et al. Perioperative hyperglycemia and risk of adverse events among patients with and without diabetes. Ann Surg 2015;261(1):97–103.

65. Duggan EW, Klopman MA, Berry AJ, et al. The Emory University perioperative algorithm for the management of hyperglycemia and diabetes in non-cardiac surgery patients. Curr Diab Rep 2016;16(3):34.

66. Garg R, Grover A, McGurk S, et al. Predictors of hyperglycemia after cardiac surgery in nondiabetic patients. J Thorac Cardiovasc Surg 2013;145(4):1083–7.

67. Underwood P, Askari R, Hurwitz S, et al. Preoperative A1C and clinical outcomes in patients with diabetes undergoing major noncardiac surgical procedures. Diabetes Care 2014;37(3):611–6.

68. American Diabetes Association. 14. Diabetes care in the hospital. Diabetes Care 2017;40(Suppl 1):S120–s127.

69. Griesdale DE, de Souza RJ, van Dam RM, et al. Intensive insulin therapy and mortality among critically ill patients: a meta-analysis including NICE-SUGAR study data. CMAJ 2009;180(8):821–7.
70. Jacobi J, Bircher N, Krinsley J, et al. Guidelines for the use of an insulin infusion for the management of hyperglycemia in critically ill patients. Crit Care Med 2012;40(12):3251–76.
71. Wenzel JT, Schwenk ES, Baratta JL, et al. Managing opioid-tolerant patients in the perioperative surgical home. Anesthesiol Clin 2016;34(2):287–301.
72. Walters TL, Mariano ER, Clark JD. Perioperative surgical home and the integral role of pain medicine. Pain Med 2015;16(9):1666–72.
73. Vetter TR, Kain ZN. Role of the perioperative surgical home in optimizing the perioperative use of opioids. Anesth Analg 2017;125(5):1653–7.
74. Upp J, Kent M, Tighe PJ. The evolution and practice of acute pain medicine. Pain Med 2013;14(1):124–44.
75. Kharasch ED, Brunt LM. Perioperative opioids and public health. Anesthesiology 2016;124(4):960–5.
76. Dowell D, Haegerich TM, Chou R. CDC guideline for prescribing opioids for chronic pain–United States, 2016. JAMA 2016;315(15):1624–45.
77. American Society of Anesthesiologists (ASA). Practice guidelines for acute pain management in the perioperative setting: an updated report by the American Society of Anesthesiologists task force on acute pain management. Anesthesiology 2012;116(2):248–73.
78. Chou R, Gordon DB, de Leon-Casasola OA, et al. Management of postoperative pain: a clinical practice guideline from the American Pain Society, the American Society of Regional Anesthesia and Pain Medicine, and the American Society of Anesthesiologists' Committee on Regional Anesthesia, Executive Committee, and Administrative Council. J Pain 2016;17(2):131–57.
79. Carli F, Scheede-Bergdahl C. Prehabilitation to enhance perioperative care. Anesthesiol Clin 2015;33(1):17–33.
80. Gillis C, Li C, Lee L, et al. Prehabilitation versus rehabilitation: a randomized control trial in patients undergoing colorectal resection for cancer. Anesthesiology 2014;121(5):937–47.
81. Partridge JS, Harari D, Dhesi JK. Frailty in the older surgical patient: a review. Age Ageing 2012;41(2):142–7.
82. Beggs T, Sepehri A, Szwajcer A, et al. Frailty and perioperative outcomes: a narrative review. Can J Anaesth 2015;62(2):143–57.
83. Dasgupta M, Rolfson DB, Stolee P, et al. Frailty is associated with postoperative complications in older adults with medical problems. Arch Gerontol Geriatr 2009;48(1):78–83.
84. Nielsen PR, Jorgensen LD, Dahl B, et al. Prehabilitation and early rehabilitation after spinal surgery: randomized clinical trial. Clin Rehabil 2010;24(2):137–48.
85. Barberan-Garcia A, Ubre M, Roca J, et al. Personalised prehabilitation in high-risk patients undergoing elective major abdominal surgery: a randomized blinded controlled trial. Ann Surg 2018;267(1):50–6.
86. Calatayud J, Casana J, Ezzatvar Y, et al. High-intensity preoperative training improves physical and functional recovery in the early post-operative periods after total knee arthroplasty: a randomized controlled trial. Knee Surg Sports Traumatol Arthrosc 2017;25(9):2864–72.
87. Santa Mina D, Clarke H, Ritvo P, et al. Effect of total-body prehabilitation on postoperative outcomes: a systematic review and meta-analysis. Physiotherapy 2014;100(3):196–207.

88. Wang L, Lee M, Zhang Z, et al. Does preoperative rehabilitation for patients planning to undergo joint replacement surgery improve outcomes? A systematic review and meta-analysis of randomised controlled trials. BMJ Open 2016;6(2): e009857.

89. Bruns ER, van den Heuvel B, Buskens CJ, et al. The effects of physical prehabilitation in elderly patients undergoing colorectal surgery: a systematic review. Colorectal Dis 2016;18(8):O267–77.

90. Cabilan CJ, Hines S, Munday J. The impact of prehabilitation on postoperative functional status, healthcare utilization, pain, and quality of life: a systematic review. Orthop Nurs 2016;35(4):224–37.

91. Nielsen PR, Andreasen J, Asmussen M, et al. Costs and quality of life for prehabilitation and early rehabilitation after surgery of the lumbar spine. BMC Health Serv Res 2008;8:209.

92. Le Roy B, Slim K. Is prehabilitation limited to preoperative exercise? Surgery 2017;162(1):192.

93. Minnella EM, Bousquet-Dion G, Awasthi R, et al. Multimodal prehabilitation improves functional capacity before and after colorectal surgery for cancer: a five-year research experience. Acta Oncol 2017;56(2):295–300.

94. Li C, Carli F, Lee L, et al. Impact of a trimodal prehabilitation program on functional recovery after colorectal cancer surgery: a pilot study. Surg Endosc 2013; 27(4):1072–82.

95. Minnella EM, Awasthi R, Gillis C, et al. Patients with poor baseline walking capacity are most likely to improve their functional status with multimodal prehabilitation. Surgery 2016;160(4):1070–9.

96. Snowden CP, Prentis JM, Anderson HL, et al. Submaximal cardiopulmonary exercise testing predicts complications and hospital length of stay in patients undergoing major elective surgery. Ann Surg 2010;251(3):535–41.

97. Levett DZ, Grocott MP. Cardiopulmonary exercise testing, prehabilitation, and Enhanced Recovery After Surgery (ERAS). Can J Anaesth 2015;62(2):131–42.

98. Carli F, Charlebois P, Stein B, et al. Randomized clinical trial of prehabilitation in colorectal surgery. Br J Surg 2010;97(8):1187–97.

99. Gillis C, Carli F. Promoting perioperative metabolic and nutritional care. Anesthesiology 2015;123(6):1455–72.

100. Kamath AF, McAuliffe CL, Kosseim LM, et al. Malnutrition in joint arthroplasty: prospective study indicates risk of unplanned ICU admission. Arch Bone Jt Surg 2016;4(2):128–31.

101. Kamath AF, Nelson CL, Elkassabany N, et al. Low albumin is a risk factor for complications after revision total knee arthroplasty. J Knee Surg 2017;30(3): 269–75.

102. Gupta R, Gan TJ. Preoperative nutrition and prehabilitation. Anesthesiol Clin 2016;34(1):143–53.

103. Sun Z, Kong XJ, Jing X, et al. Nutritional risk screening 2002 as a predictor of postoperative outcomes in patients undergoing abdominal surgery: a systematic review and meta-analysis of prospective cohort studies. PLoS One 2015; 10(7):e0132857.

104. Isenring E, Elia M. Which screening method is appropriate for older cancer patients at risk for malnutrition? Nutrition 2015;31(4):594–7.

105. Weimann A, Braga M, Carli F, et al. ESPEN guideline: clinical nutrition in surgery. Clin Nutr 2017;36(3):623–50.

106. Tsimopoulou I, Pasquali S, Howard R, et al. Psychological prehabilitation before cancer surgery: a systematic review. Ann Surg Oncol 2015;22(13):4117–23.

107. Le Roy B, Selvy M, Slim K. The concept of prehabilitation: what the surgeon needs to know? J Visc Surg 2016;153(2):109–12.

108. Chen BP, Awasthi R, Sweet SN, et al. Four-week prehabilitation program is sufficient to modify exercise behaviors and improve preoperative functional walking capacity in patients with colorectal cancer. Support Care Cancer 2017;25(1):33–40.

109. Sisko AM, Keehan SP, Cuckler GA, et al. National health expenditure projections, 2013-23: faster growth expected with expanded coverage and improving economy. Health Aff (Millwood) 2014;33(10):1841–50.

110. Lee TH, Marcantonio ER, Mangione CM, et al. Derivation and prospective validation of a simple index for prediction of cardiac risk of major noncardiac surgery. Circulation 1999;100(10):1043–9.

111. Davis C, Tait G, Carroll J, et al. The Revised Cardiac Risk Index in the new millennium: a single-centre prospective cohort re-evaluation of the original variables in 9,519 consecutive elective surgical patients. Can J Anaesth 2013;60(9): 855–63.

112. Ford MK, Beattie WS, Wijeysundera DN. Systematic review: prediction of perioperative cardiac complications and mortality by the revised cardiac risk index. Ann Intern Med 2010;152(1):26–35.

113. Gupta PK, Gupta H, Sundaram A, et al. Development and validation of a risk calculator for prediction of cardiac risk after surgery. Circulation 2011;124(4): 381–7.

114. Caprini JA. Risk assessment as a guide for the prevention of the many faces of venous thromboembolism. Am J Surg 2010;199(1 Suppl):S3–10.

115. U.S. Agency for Healthcare Research and Quality. Chapter 4. Choose the model to assess VTE and bleeding risk. 2016. Available at: http://www.ahrq.gov/professionals/quality-patient-safety/patient-safety-resources/resources/vtguide/vtguide4.html. Accessed October 15, 2017.

116. Jenkins IH, White RH, Amin AN, et al. Reducing the incidence of hospital-associated venous thromboembolism within a network of academic hospitals: findings from five University of California medical centers. J Hosp Med 2016; 11(Suppl 2):S22–s28.

117. Parvizi J, Huang R, Raphael IJ, et al. Symptomatic pulmonary embolus after joint arthroplasty: stratification of risk factors. Clin Orthop Relat Res 2014;472(3): 903–12.

118. Nagappa M, Wong J, Singh M, et al. An update on the various practical applications of the STOP-Bang questionnaire in anesthesia, surgery, and perioperative medicine. Curr Opin Anaesthesiol 2017;30(1):118–25.

119. Nagappa M, Patra J, Wong J, et al. Association of STOP-bang questionnaire as a screening tool for sleep apnea and postoperative complications: a systematic review and bayesian meta-analysis of prospective and retrospective cohort studies. Anesth Analg 2017;125(4):1301–8.

120. Kroenke K, Spitzer RL, Williams JB, et al. The patient health questionnaire somatic, anxiety, and depressive symptom scales: a systematic review. Gen Hosp Psychiatry 2010;32(4):345–59.

121. Thombs BD, Benedetti A, Kloda LA, et al. The diagnostic accuracy of the patient health questionnaire-2 (PHQ-2), patient health questionnaire-8 (PHQ-8), and patient health questionnaire-9 (PHQ-9) for detecting major depression: protocol for a systematic review and individual patient data meta-analyses. Syst Rev 2014;3:124.

122. Spitzer RL, Kroenke K, Williams JB, et al. A brief measure for assessing generalized anxiety disorder: the GAD-7. Arch Intern Med 2006;166(10): 1092–7.
123. Plummer F, Manea L, Trepel D, et al. Screening for anxiety disorders with the GAD-7 and GAD-2: a systematic review and diagnostic metaanalysis. Gen Hosp Psychiatry 2016;39:24–31.
124. Borson S, Scanlan JM, Chen P, et al. The Mini-Cog as a screen for dementia: validation in a population-based sample. J Am Geriatr Soc 2003;51(10): 1451–4.
125. Dworkin A, Lee DS, An AR, et al. A simple tool to predict development of delirium after elective surgery. J Am Geriatr Soc 2016;64(11):e149–53.
126. Hill J, McVay JM, Walter-Ginzburg A, et al. Validation of a brief screen for cognitive impairment (BSCI) administered by telephone for use in the Medicare population. Dis Manag 2005;8(4):223–34.
127. Fillit H, Mohs RC, Lewis BE, et al. A brief telephonic instrument to screen for cognitive impairment in a managed care population. J Clin Outcomes Manag 2003;10(8):419–29.
128. Castanho TC, Amorim L, Zihl J, et al. Telephone-based screening tools for mild cognitive impairment and dementia in aging studies: a review of validated instruments. Front Aging Neurosci 2014;6:16.
129. Rolfson DB, Majumdar SR, Tsuyuki RT, et al. Validity and reliability of the Edmonton Frail Scale. Age Ageing 2006;35(5):526–9.
130. Hyder JA, Wakeam E, Habermann EB, et al. Derivation and validation of a simple calculator to predict home discharge after surgery. J Am Coll Surg 2014; 218(2):226–36.
131. Oldmeadow LB, McBurney H, Robertson VJ. Predicting risk of extended inpatient rehabilitation after hip or knee arthroplasty. J Arthroplasty 2003;18(6): 775–9.
132. Oldmeadow LB, McBurney H, Robertson VJ, et al. Targeted postoperative care improves discharge outcome after hip or knee arthroplasty. Arch Phys Med Rehabil 2004;85(9):1424–7.
133. Ewing JA. Detecting alcoholism. The CAGE questionnaire. JAMA 1984;252(14): 1905–7.
134. Ewing JA. Screening for alcoholism using CAGE. Cut down, annoyed, guilty, eye opener. JAMA 1998;280(22):1904–5.
135. Bradley KA, Bush KR, McDonell MB, et al. Screening for problem drinking : comparison of CAGE and AUDIT. J Gen Intern Med 1998;13(6):379–88.
136. Bradley KA, DeBenedetti AF, Volk RJ, et al. AUDIT-C as a brief screen for alcohol misuse in primary care. Alcohol Clin Exp Res 2007;31(7):1208–17.
137. McAnally HB. Opioid dependence risk factors and risk assessment. Opioid dependence. Cham (Switzerland): Springer; 2017. p. 233–64.
138. Webster LR, Webster RM. Predicting aberrant behaviors in opioid-treated patients: preliminary validation of the Opioid Risk Tool. Pain Med 2005;6(6): 432–42.
139. Butler SF, Fernandez K, Benoit C, et al. Validation of the revised Screener and Opioid Assessment for Patients with Pain (SOAPP-R). J Pain 2008;9(4): 360–72.
140. Butler SF, Budman SH, Fernandez KC, et al. Cross-validation of a Screener to Predict Opioid Misuse in Chronic Pain Patients (SOAPP-R). J Addict Med 2009;3(2):66–73.

141. Finkelman MD, Smits N, Kulich RJ, et al. Development of short-form versions of the Screener and Opioid Assessment for Patients with Pain-Revised (SOAPP-R): a proof-of-principle study. Pain Med 2017;18(7):1292–302.

142. Black RA, McCaffrey SA, Villapiano AJ, et al. Development and validation of an eight-item brief form of the SOAPP-R (SOAPP-8). Pain Med 2017. [Epub ahead of print].

Perioperative Surgical Home for the Patient with Chronic Pain

Talal W. Khan, MD, MBA*, Smith Manion, MD

KEYWORDS

- Perioperative surgical home • Chronic pain
- Perioperative management of chronic pain • Multimodal analgesia • Opioid epidemic
- Perioperative considerations for the opioid epidemic

KEY POINTS

- Perioperative management of the patient with chronic pain is complex and expensive.
- The perioperative surgical home provides an optimal framework for the management of the patient with chronic pain.
- Multimodal analgesia is a key consideration for management of the complexities associated with chronic pain throughout the perioperative continuum.
- Preoperative patient assessment and optimization, intraoperative multimodal, opioid-sparing analgesia, postoperative management and care coordination, and postdischarge transitions of care are essential components of the perioperative surgical home.

INTRODUCTION

The delivery of health care in the United States continues to face many challenges with rising costs and a growing body of evidence indicating uneven quality.[1] An aging population, increasing medical comorbidities, and a demand for the latest procedures with no regard to cost or outcomes continues to compound the issue. Our current model of surgical and procedural care is fragmented and associated with wide variability, not only in cost, but also quality.[2] In recognition of the fact that anesthesiologists are at the forefront of coordination and delivery of perioperative care, the American Society of Anesthesiologists has declared support for a paradigm shift in perioperative care, which is now widely known as the perioperative surgical home (PSH).[3] Additionally, chronic pain affects more than 100 million Americans at a cost of approximately $635 billion.[4] These patients also require surgical and procedural care. The

Disclosure Statement: The authors have no relevant disclosures.
Department of Anesthesiology and Pain Medicine, University of Kansas Medical Center, 3901 Rainbow Boulevard, MS 1034, Kansas City, KS 66160, USA
* Corresponding author.
E-mail address: tkhan@kumc.edu

PSH framework provides an ideal model for the management of this complex patient population from the decision for surgery to preoperative assessment and optimization, intraoperative care, inpatient postsurgical management, and transitions after discharge.

OVERVIEW OF THE PERIOPERATIVE SURGICAL HOME

The PSH has been described as a patient-centered approach to the surgical patient with a strong emphasis on process standardization, evidence-based clinical care pathways, and coordinated and integrated care. This model of care helps the patient and their family members to navigate the complexities of the perioperative continuum from the time of decision for surgery to the postdischarge phase.[5] In a 2009 *Health Affairs* editorial, Berwick[6] defined patient-centered care as, "The experience (to the extent the informed, individual patient desires it) of transparency, individualization, recognition, respect, dignity, and choice in all matters, without exception, related to one's person, circumstances, and relationships in health care." This definition of patient-centered care, as well as the core principles of the PSH, seeks to reframe the concept of value in health care, including surgical and perioperative services, from the perspective of the patient[7,8] (**Fig. 1**).

PERIOPERATIVE MANAGEMENT OF THE PATIENT WITH CHRONIC PAIN

It is estimated that 100 million Americans suffer from chronic pain; this astounding number surpasses the combination of diabetes, heart disease, and cancer combined. Studies show that 15% to more than 50% of patients presenting for surgery in the United States consume opioids chronically.[9] The American health care system is currently coping with both an opioid epidemic and a chronic pain epidemic. Consequently, the volume of patients undergoing surgery who have concomitant chronic pain issues and/or opioid use is escalating. It is, therefore, imperative to understand how best to optimize the perioperative management of chronic pain and opioid-tolerant patients, thereby enhancing patient care and lessening the socioeconomic burden.

Chronic pain and opioid-tolerant patients are at risk for inadequate perioperative analgesia for multiple reasons. The US Food and Drug Administration has defined the opioid-tolerant patient as anyone who has used opioids for 7 days or longer (**Box 1**). Practitioners need to be cognizant of this issue, because the neuroendocrine stress response to uncontrolled acute pain can have significant sequelae. These consequences include an increased risk of myocardial ischemia, impaired respiratory function resulting in hypoxemia and pneumonia, increased incidence of deep vein thrombosis and thromboembolism, decreased gastrointestinal motility, decreased immune function, and poor wound healing (**Fig. 2**).

PATIENT IDENTIFICATION

Chronic pain and opioid-tolerant patients require early and aggressive interventions to modify the postsurgical pain trajectory. Anesthesiologists and surgeons need to implement systems to identify chronic pain and opioid-tolerant patients days before surgery and not just minutes before the procedure. Such a process allows care providers sufficient time to:

1. Assess the patient's pain location and any functional impairment that may compromise surgery, perioperative care, or rehabilitative efforts;
2. Query the current pain medication regimen;

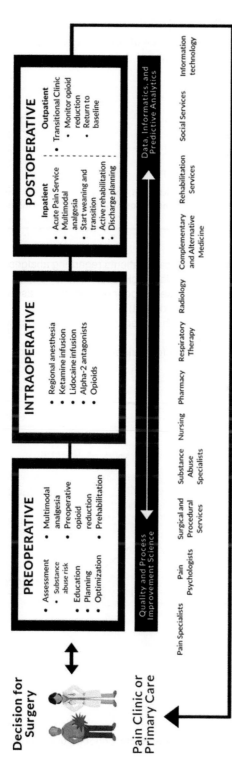

Fig. 1. The perioperative surgical home for the patient with chronic pain.

Box 1
US Food and Drug Administration definition of an opioid-tolerant patient

Seven or more days of opioid use, including

- 60 mg oral morphine per day;
- 25 µg transdermal fentanyl per hour;
- 30 mg oral oxycodone per day;
- 8 mg oral hydromorphone per day;
- 25 mg oral oxymorphone per day; or
- An equianalgesic dose of any other opioid.

Data from US Food and Drug Administration. Extended-release (ER) and long-acting (LA) opioid analgesics risk evaluation and mitigation strategy (REMS). Washington, DC: US Food and Drug Administration; 2012.

---

3. Establish indications for and educate patients regarding analgesic options, such as peripheral nerve block or neuraxial blockade;
4. Identify psychological factors linked to poor outcomes and assuage fears and anxiety related to postoperative discomfort;
5. Optimize surgical decisions such as technique, incision location, and expertise; and
6. Formulate an individualized plan for perioperative pain control.

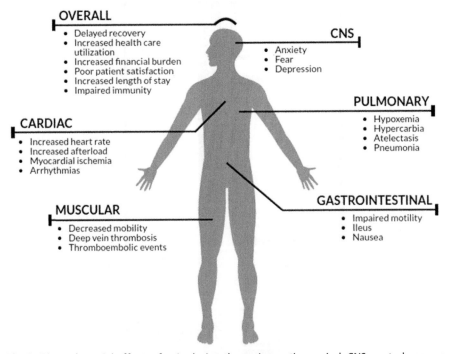

Fig. 2. Biopsychosocial effects of pain during the perioperative period. CNS, central nervous system.

A crucial factor throughout perioperative patient education is to establish appropriate and realistic expectations with regard to the postoperative pain experience, including pain with movement, adverse effects of medication, and the anticipated duration of analgesic usage involved in the normal healing process. Uniquely tailored educational, rehabilitation, and perioperative analgesic plans are associated with reduced postoperative opioid consumption, less preoperative anxiety, fewer requests for sedative medications, and a shortened duration of stay after surgery.[10]

In assessing the preoperative analgesic regimen, it is important to arrive at an accurate portrayal of the patient's pain regimen, including any misuse of prescribed medication or illicit drug use, to establish a more accurate perioperative plan. If significant misuse such as addiction or diversion is suspected, a conversation among providers will help to determine whether interventions are necessary before surgery to optimize outcomes.

Providers should inquire about the prescriber, exact medication dosage, route of administration, schedule, and when the last dose of medication was used. At times, practitioners may need to contact prescribers and pharmacies directly to verify the patient's preoperative regimen. Patients engaged in collaborative care, including shared decision making with practitioners, have been shown to experience better overall health-related outcomes.[10]

PREOPERATIVE ASSESSMENT AND OPTIMIZATION

Because chronic pain and opioid-tolerant patients have such challenging postoperative pain experiences, it is imperative to initiate a preventative, multimodal treatment approach (**Table 1**). Multimodal analgesic techniques have been useful to target pain along various pathways involving transduction, transmission, modulation, and perception by the central nervous system to assist in acute pain control and also in an attempt to prevent neural sensitization leading to possible persistent postoperative pain. Providers need to review patient comorbidities such as renal, pulmonary, or liver insufficiency; the potential for perioperative blood loss or coagulopathy; need for bone healing; and the anticipated surgical positioning. Although no panacea exists, many preoperative adjuncts are available, including medications, physical or cognitive therapies, and injections. The current literature supports regional anesthesia and analgesia, nonsteroidal antiinflammatory drugs (NSAIDs), acetaminophen, and gabapentinoids as the most successful preemptive therapies.

Strong evidence demonstrates the benefits of site-specific peripheral nerve or neuraxial blockade as a component of perioperative analgesia for the opioid-tolerant patient.[11] Individuals undergoing upper or lower extremity surgical procedures will benefit from a single-shot peripheral nerve blockade with a long-acting local anesthetic. The addition of clonidine or dexamethasone can prolong the duration of the blockade.[12] Continuous peripheral nerve blockade with perineural catheter placement for prolonged analgesia has been shown to decrease postsurgical pain with a decreased reliance on opioid therapy, accelerated resumption of physical therapy, fewer sleep disturbances, and augmented patient satisfaction.[13] Local wound infiltration has been shown to be successful for arthroscopic knee surgery, total knee arthroplasty, laparotomy, and hemorrhoid surgery, and may be considered when nerve blockade is not viable. Thoracic epidural analgesia has been shown to be superior to systemic opioid therapy in a variety of thoracic and upper abdominal surgeries. Thoracic epidural analgesia can decrease the duration of mechanical ventilation by 20%, decrease the risk of pulmonary complications, decrease the duration of postoperative ileus, and may help to prevent postsurgical muscle catabolism.[14] Epidural

Table 1
Components of multimodal analgesia

	Preoperative	Intraoperative	Postoperative
Pharmacologic	Acetaminophen Nonsteroidal antiinflammatory drugs Cyclooxygenase-2 inhibitor Gabapentinoid Glucocorticoid Tramadol Oral N-methyl-D-aspartate Inhibitor Alpha2-adrenergic receptor inhibitor	Ketamine IV/infusion Opioid IV/infusion Lidocaine infusion	Acetaminophen Nonsteroidal antiinflammatory drugs Gabapentinoid Ketamine infusion Lidocaine infusion Tramadol Opioid (PCA)/oral
Nonpharmacologic	TENS Cognitive modalities	Local anesthetic infiltration Intraarticular/periarticular injection Regional anesthetic techniques Neuraxial anesthetic techniques	Continuous catheter techniques Local anesthetic infiltration TENS Cognitive modalities Neurostimulation techniques[41]
Self-management	Breathing techniques Distraction Positive thought Exercise Manage stress/anxiety Sleep Eat healthy Pace activities		Breathing techniques Distraction Positive thought Exercise Manage stress/anxiety Sleep Eat healthy Pace activities

Abbreviations: IV, intravenous; PCA, patient-controlled analgesia; TENS, transcutaneous electrical stimulation.

analgesia has a well-established safety profile, although hypotension can limit the use of neuraxial local anesthetic. If hypotension or coagulopathy are of significant concern, paravertebral or transverse abdominis plane blockade are practical options, especially if unilateral analgesia is desired.

The use of the cyclooxygenase-2 inhibitor, celecoxib, or acetaminophen in conjunction with opioids has demonstrated decreased perioperative analgesic requirements compared with opioids alone. Celecoxib has gained significant popularity for presurgical use given its lack of platelet inhibition, but it can compromise renal function and is contraindicated in patients after coronary artery bypass graft surgery. Celecoxib doses most frequently used are 200 to 400 mg approximately 1 hour before surgery. In contrast with celecoxib, acetaminophen has weak antiinflammatory properties and primarily works as a centrally acting analgesic. Acetaminophen 1000 mg has been shown to be successful via an oral route, although a rectal suppository is a viable but less desirable route of administration. Intravenous administration of NSAIDs or acetaminophen may have faster onset, but there is no apparent clinical benefit compared with the oral route and it incurs a much higher cost.

The 2 gabapentinoids predominantly used perioperatively are gabapentin and pregabalin. Both medications seem to be effective when administered preoperatively, and some studies have shown benefit in diminishing the risk of developing chronic postsurgical pain when sustained postoperatively. The ideal doses for gabapentin or pregabalin have not been well-established, but the typical gabapentin doses of 600 mg or 1200 mg preoperatively have been deemed successful. Gabapentin has less systemic absorption compared with pregabalin, especially at escalating doses, and thus pregabalin at 150 mg or 300 mg may be better suited for preoperative use given its superior bioavailability and potentially lower side effect profile, albeit at an additional cost. There is evidence the combination of cyclooxygenase-2 inhibitor with acetaminophen and a gabapentinoid is superior to monotherapy alone, and such a triad should be strongly considered for the patient with chronic pain or opioid-tolerant pain before undergoing major surgery.

Complementary therapies such as cognitive behavioral therapy should also be considered as part of a multimodal approach in high-risk adults. There is insufficient evidence to recommend one specific technique, but guided imagery and some relaxation methods have shown promise, although they frequently require patient engagement in preoperative training for optimal results.[10]

Conventional preoperative education for the opioid-tolerant pain patient is to maintain the preoperative opioid regimen unchanged, including on the day of surgery. Concerns with minimizing opioids before surgery include medication withdrawal and increased discomfort and distress preceding a surgical insult. However, this conventional therapy needs to be further analyzed. It is evident that opioid-tolerant patients have a more challenging postoperative course. A superior method would be to reduce or omit opioid consumption for a sufficient period of time before any major procedure, thereby minimizing any concurrent hyperalgesia and resensitizing the patient to perioperative analgesics. The need for high-dose opioid regimens postoperatively and associated adverse effects could theoretically also be diminished. Some existing evidence supports this concept in total joint arthroplasty, where patients who decreased opioid use by 50% before surgery had significantly higher physical component scores compared with the opioid-dependent group and had similar outcomes compared with the opioid-naïve cohort.[15] Preoperative opioid reduction may prove to be an important and easily modifiable risk factor, and needs to be explored.

INTRAOPERATIVE MANAGEMENT

Adequate preoperative assessment will help providers to prepare for and enact intraoperative management plans. No difference in the postoperative pain experience has been demonstrated between general anesthesia sustained by volatile anesthetics versus propofol infusion. However, specific infusion therapies do seem to augment analgesia in the patient with chronic pain.

Ketamine

Ketamine is perhaps the most supported therapy for the opioid-tolerant patient. Ketamine antagonizes the N-methyl-D-aspartate receptor but also decreases central excitability, decreases acute postoperative opiate tolerance, and may modulate opioid receptors. Loftus and colleagues[16] performed a randomized controlled trial in opiate-tolerant patients (30 mg oral morphine equivalents or more) undergoing major spine surgery. A ketamine 0.5 mg/kg bolus on induction followed by a 10 µg/kg/min intraoperative infusion stopped at wound closure significantly reduced total morphine consumption at 24 hours, 48 hours, and even at 6 weeks with decreased pain intensity immediately after surgery and again at 6 weeks. No significant side effects from ketamine were reported, although hallucinations and nightmares may occur. Relative contradictions to ketamine include schizophrenia, an overactive sympathomimetic disease process, and significantly elevated intracranial pressure.

Alpha-2 Agonists

Alpha-2 adrenergic agonists act at the dorsal horn of the spinal cord to reduce pain but also possess sedative, anxiolytic, and potentially antiemetic properties with minimal risk of respiratory depression. The use of alpha-2 agonists can be associated with hypotension, bradycardia, and dose-dependent sedation. Dexmedetomidine has been shown to minimize opioid use in the short term in patients undergoing laparoscopic bariatric surgery and total abdominal hysterectomy, but no long-term benefit has been established. A Cochrane review showed that dexmedetomidine reduces intraoperative opioid consumption compared with placebo but does not significantly affect pain scores. Clonidine seems to strengthen the opioid effect and may counteract the development of opioid tolerance. Dexmedetomidine and clonidine, when administered perioperatively, can reduce morphine consumption up to 24 hours and to a similar extent as acetaminophen, but not as much as other NSAIDs.[17] Alpha-2 agonists have not been specifically studied in chronic pain and opioid-tolerant patients, but should be considered as an integral aspect of a multimodal approach.

Intravenous Lidocaine

Lidocaine is a local anesthetic that can provide analgesia when used intravenously. Its mechanism of action is likely multifactorial, with both peripheral and central effects. Lidocaine has been shown to reduce the inflammatory response to tissue ischemia and attenuate the tissue damage induced by endothelial and vascular cytokines through a mechanism involving the release of adenosine triphosphate and K^+ channels.[18] Perioperative and intraoperative lidocaine infusions have been studied in both laparoscopic and open abdominal operations. Intravenous lidocaine resulted in a shorter duration of ileus, improved quality of analgesia for 48 hours, earlier rehabilitation, and decreased duration of stay. A common regimen is a 2 mg/kg bolus followed by a 2 mg/kg/h infusion with dose adjustment performed in patients with hepatic insufficiency.

Opioids

The optimal intraoperative opioid regimen for the opioid-tolerant patient has not been defined. It is common practice for providers to escalate intraoperative opioid dosage or maintain continuous opioid infusions with greater steady-state plasma levels in the opioid-tolerant patient. However, there is evidence that intravenous opioids can quickly cause a pronociceptive environment with high-dose intraoperative opioids actually precipitating hyperalgesia with increased postoperative pain intensity and opioid requirements.[19] Further, it has been demonstrated that oral opioid rotation can improve analgesic quality and decrease undesirable side effects in 2 of 3 patients postoperatively, likely through incomplete cross-tolerance of the agents used.[20] Although the best intraoperative regimen remains unclear, the practice of minimizing or rotating intraoperative opioids while under general anesthesia and assessing analgesic outcomes needs to be explored.

POSTOPERATIVE MANAGEMENT

The in-hospital management of chronic pain and opioid-tolerant patients can be a challenging clinical scenario and frequently requires a multidisciplinary approach.

In designing and executing a postoperative analgesic plan, certain goals need to be entertained:

1. Instilling a sense of control to the patient;
2. Enabling early mobilization and optimizing analgesia to achieve functional milestones;
3. Attenuating the perioperative stress response; and
4. Accelerating recovery and decreasing the duration of hospitalization.

Multimodal analgesic techniques need to be used routinely in chronic pain and opioid-tolerant patients, because they have been shown to increase patient satisfaction and decrease opioid consumption, opioid-related adverse effects, postoperative pain, and postanesthesia care unit and hospital durations of stay.[21] It is also critical to appreciate that patients with chronic pain consistently start with and maintain higher reported pain scores compared with opioid-naïve individuals and are subject to an increased risk of opioid-related adverse effects. In the absence of contraindications, the patient with chronic pain should routinely receive a scheduled NSAID, acetaminophen, and a gabapentinoid after major surgery. Gabapentin was associated with a statistically significant decrease in postoperative pain at 24 hours and less postoperative analgesic use compared with control.[22] A metaanalysis of pregabalin demonstrated decreased cumulative opioid consumption at 24 hours with lower risk of opioid-related adverse effects such as vomiting.[23] Ketamine infusions in the postoperative arena have been shown to be safe and may offer some advantage in the complex patient.[24]

It is recommended that, unless contraindicated, patients receive oral opioid therapy as soon as possible postoperatively. Intravenous patient-controlled analgesia can be helpful during the first 24 to 48 hours after extensive surgeries and in assessing a 24-hour oral morphine equivalent before transitioning to an oral regimen. Oxycodone is typically preferred over hydrocodone, because hydrocodone needs to be converted to hydromorphone to achieve analgesia. A liberal oral opioid regimen may help to improve functional restoration and decrease the duration of stay; after hospital discharge, the oral regimen can be monitored and weaned as the healing process progresses.

POSTOPERATIVE PAIN CONTINUUM

Involved decision making throughout the entire perioperative process, rather than just the prehospital or in-hospital components, is critical to making high-value contributions. For the chronic pain and opioid-tolerant patients, the time after hospital discharge is frequently the most challenging. It is not uncommon for postoperative opioid tapering to require more than a month. Furthermore, the patient with chronic pain is likely a part of a subgroup at risk for developing chronic postsurgical pain. Psychological comorbidities such as depression, anxiety, and catastrophizing are risk factors for chronic postsurgical pain, and studies have shown that 60% of patients with chronic pain report psychological comorbidities. Perioperative teams need to maintain the ability to follow patients by phone, secure e-mail, or even in a clinic setting for up to a few months with the goal of stabilizing or weaning analgesics and enabling rehabilitation and early return to work.[9]

A multidisciplinary transitional pain clinic would be ideal to address the complexities of the chronic pain and opioid-tolerant patient after surgical intervention. It is unrealistic for primary care physicians to be responsible for managing such complexities of postsurgical care. Transitional pain clinic practitioners could manage perineural catheter infusions, closely monitor and adjust necessary analgesics, help to mitigate psychosocial burdens, and facilitate the secure return of unused opioid prescriptions.

PERIOPERATIVE CONSIDERATIONS FOR PATIENTS WITH INTRATHECAL DRUG DELIVERY SYSTEMS AND SPINAL CORD STIMULATORS
Perioperative Management of the Patient with Intrathecal Drug Delivery Systems

Intrathecal drug delivery systems (IDDS) are increasingly used for the management of refractory cancer pain and non–cancer-related pain.[25] Patients with IDDS who are referred for perioperative management of an unrelated surgical problem present unique challenges. Despite the prevalence of these devices, the literature on perioperative management of patients with IDDS is sparse and recommendations or consensus statements from major pain societies do not exist.[26] Concerns around the perioperative period may include respiratory depression, excessive sedation, feasibility of regional anesthetic techniques, and postoperative analgesia. Grider and colleagues[26] recommend the following:

1. Devices should be interrogated before and after surgery, even though electrocautery does not interfere with IDDS;
2. Intrathecal infusion should be continued throughout the perioperative period because an abrupt cessation of intrathecal baclofen can be life threatening;
3. The continuation of intrathecal analgesia maintains baseline analgesic requirements and can be supplemented with oral or intravenous opioids for incisional pain;
4. Multimodal analgesia should be used, because many of these patients may be opioid tolerant; and
5. The course of the intrathecal catheter should be determined before surgery or regional anesthesia to protect the integrity of the catheter.

Ziconotide, a first-tier drug for intrathecal therapy that has been approved by the US Food and Drug Administration, is a selective N-type calcium channel inhibitor.[27] Side effects of this agent that require special consideration during the perioperative period include postural hypotension, confusion, agitation, and nausea.[28] Patel and colleagues[28] note that hypotension from ziconotide can be exacerbated by the induction and maintenance of general anesthesia secondary to the vasodilatory effects of intravenous and inhaled anesthetic agents. One strategy to help mitigate this risk might be to gradually reduce and eventually eliminate ziconotide around the perioperative period. Other strategies should include maintenance of vascular volume and peripheral vascular resistance through avoidance of beta-blockade and continuation of clear liquids up to 2 hours before induction.[28]

Perioperative Management of the Patient with Spinal Cord Stimulators

Spinal cord stimulators (SCS) are minimally invasive, reversible modalities that are being increasingly used earlier in the treatment algorithm for various pain conditions, including chronic back pain, lumbar radicular pain, postlaminectomy syndromes, complex regional pain syndrome, and various other neuropathic pain states.[29] Conventional SCS treats pain by the application of electrical impulses to the dorsal column of the spinal cord to create a modification of pain perception.[30] Recent years have witnessed technical advances in the various programming parameters as well as numbers of new devices available for deployment and stimulation beyond typical dorsal column stimulation, such as dorsal root ganglion stimulation[31] and peripheral nerve stimulation. As these devices become more commonplace, anesthesia teams will be called on to evaluate and manage these patients throughout the perioperative continuum.[32]

Although there is scant literature regarding the perioperative considerations and management of patients with SCS, there are a multitude of factors that present the potential for disastrous consequences for the patient and/or the device, including the complexity of the devices themselves, implant techniques and locations, interaction with operating room equipment, and patient comorbidities. The PSH framework provides an ideal model to elucidate and address these complexities for optimal management of these complex patients. These patients should be identified during the preoperative assessment and an optimal multidisciplinary, multimodal management plan should be formulated with the assistance of the pain physician. A thorough review of patient records and discussion with the implanting physician will identify the device model and manufacturer. Because each company has specific labeling restrictions regarding MRI compatibility, the appropriate manual should be reviewed or the patient service representative for the company should be contacted to provide the most up-to-date information. Additionally, patients presenting for an anesthetic should have their device interrogated and reprogrammed to the lowest possible amplitude and turned off before the induction of anesthesia.[33] Active SCS may interfere with electrocardiographic readings, resulting in high-frequency artifact.[34] Programming the SCS to the inactive mode will help to mitigate the risk of interference.

Monopolar electrocautery presents risks to the patient and the device. Existing SCS manufacturers recommend the avoidance of monopolar electrocautery in patients with SCS implants. If electrocautery is required, bipolar electrocautery is recommended. The grounding pad should be placed as far away as possible from the SCS and on the contralateral side of the battery. The SCS system should be interrogated after the procedure to ensure adequate impedance and confirm that there has been no damage to the system before reactivation of stimulation.[32]

Although the risks for an adverse interaction between SCS and pacemakers, implantable cardiac defibrillators, and other implanted cardiovascular electronic devices exist, a number of reports support safe simultaneous use of these devices.[33] A detailed discussion with the patient and cardiologist will help to weigh the risks and benefits of the concomitant use of these devices, leading to an informed decision. The interaction between the devices can also be tested intraoperatively with the implantable cardiovascular device set at maximal sensitivity and SCS at maximally tolerated stimulation parameters.[35]

Parturients with SCS should be referred to the obstetric anesthesia service or preanesthesia assessment clinics early to plan analgesia and possible anesthesia for the peripartum phase. A discussion with the patient and the chronic pain physician will help to identify the type of device and level of placement. Generally, percutaneous SCS leads are advanced into the epidural at the lower thoracic or upper lumbar levels with the tips located in the T6 to T10 region. This placement allows for safe epidural catheter placement or intrathecal access at the lower lumbar levels. The risk of patchy epidural analgesia owing to fibrous tissue development in the upper lumbar and lower thoracic regions still exists.[33] Although no harm to the mother or baby has been reported, SCS use during pregnancy should only be continued after a thorough review of the risks and benefits with the patient and the obstetrician.[36]

PERIOPERATIVE MANAGEMENT OF THE PATIENT ON THERAPY FOR OPIOID USE DISORDER

The increase of opioid-related deaths and the recognition of opioid use disorder have necessitated medication-assisted treatment for this condition. Along with counseling and support, medications commonly used for the treatment of opioid use disorder include methadone (a μ-receptor agonist and N-methyl-D-aspartate antagonist), buprenorphine (a partial agonist at the μ-receptor and an antagonist at the κ and Δ receptors), and naltrexone (a μ and κ receptor antagonist).

The main concerns in this patient population during the perioperative period include inadequate analgesia, drug overdose, and withdrawal. Methadone is about 3 times more bioavailable than morphine, with an onset of action within 60 minutes of oral ingestion. The half-life is long but unpredictable, with a range from about 8 to 60 hours and an average of about 23 hours. Its typical analgesic action lasts for about 6 to 8 hours and is commonly used on a thrice daily regimen for pain control and on a once daily regimen for opioid addiction. Concomitant use of methadone with additional drugs that prolong the QT interval can increase the risk of cardiac arrhythmia. Unless specifically contraindicated, the patient's outpatient regimen of methadone should be maintained. If a parenteral route is mandatory, methadone can be converted from an oral to an intravenous regimen at a 2:1 ratio.[37,38]

Buprenorphine is available in intravenous, sublingual, and transdermal forms. It is used for opioid use disorder as well as chronic pain.[39] The unique properties of this agent pose significant challenges for the management of acute pain, including inadequate analgesia and the risk of relapse. A review of the literature reveals limited data on the perioperative management of patients on buprenorphine. Based on case reports and expert opinion, Anderson and colleagues[40] have made suggestions for the management of buprenorphine therapy in elective and urgent and emergent cases. In elective cases, it is important to communicate with an addiction specialist or chronic pain physician to understand the goals of therapy and patient characteristics. For patients with well-controlled pain at baseline, it may be reasonable to continue buprenorphine throughout the perioperative phase while ensuring multimodal analgesia.[40] For patients being considered for elective surgery with moderate to severe baseline pain, it may be necessary to reschedule the case until a comprehensive plan can be devised with the involvement of all stakeholders, including the patient. In urgent or emergent situations for patients with moderate to severe pain, it may be necessary to discontinue buprenorphine, incorporate regional anesthesia, start patient-controlled analgesia, and maximize adjuncts including acetaminophen, antineuralgics, and dexmedetomidine. A common practice is to discontinue oral buprenorphine approximately 48 to 72 hours and transdermal buprenorphine for 7 days before surgical intervention. The patient should be followed by the acute pain service in a monitored care setting (e.g., an intensive care unit) and a challenging postoperative course should be anticipated.[40]

SUMMARY

The management of acute pain for the phenotypically distinct patient who suffers from chronic pain is challenging. The care of these patients is expensive and discordant. The physician-led, multidisciplinary, patient-centric, care coordination framework of the PSH is an optimal vehicle for the management of these patients. The engagement of physician anesthesiologists in the optimization, in-hospital management and post-discharge care of the patient with chronic pain will lead to optimal outcomes, reduced health care expenditures, and improved health in this unique patient population.

REFERENCES

1. Porter ME, Lee TH. From volume to value in health care: the work begins. JAMA 2016;316(10):1047–8.

2. Cyriac J, Cannesson M, Kain Z. Pain management and the perioperative surgical home: getting the desired outcome right. Reg Anesth Pain Med 2015;40(1):1–2.
3. Kain ZN, Vakharia S, Garson L, et al. The perioperative surgical home as a future perioperative practice model. Anesth Analg 2014;118(5):1126–30.
4. Institute of Medicine. Relieving pain in America: a blueprint for transforming prevention, care, education, and research. Washington, DC: The National Academies Press; 2011.
5. Vetter TR, Goeddel LA, Boudreaux AM, et al. The perioperative surgical home: how can it make the case so everyone wins? BMC Anesthesiol 2013;13:6.
6. Berwick DM. What 'patient-centered' should mean: confessions of an extremist. Health Aff (Millwood) 2009;28(4):w555–565.
7. Porter ME. What is value in health care? N Engl J Med 2010;363(26):2477–81.
8. Neuman MD. Patient satisfaction and value in anesthesia care. Anesthesiology 2011;114(5):1019–20.
9. Walters TL, Mariano ER, Clark JD. Perioperative surgical home and the integral role of pain medicine. Pain Med 2015;16(9):1666–72.
10. Chou R, Gordon DB, de Leon-Casasola OA, et al. Management of postoperative pain: a clinical practice guideline from the American Pain Society, the American Society of Regional Anesthesia and Pain Medicine, and the American Society of Anesthesiologists' committee on regional anesthesia, executive committee, and administrative council. J Pain 2016;17(2):131–57.
11. Humble SR, Dalton AJ, Li L. A systematic review of therapeutic interventions to reduce acute and chronic post-surgical pain after amputation, thoracotomy or mastectomy. Eur J Pain 2015;19(4):451–65.
12. Huynh TM, Marret E, Bonnet F. Combination of dexamethasone and local anaesthetic solution in peripheral nerve blocks: a meta-analysis of randomised controlled trials. Eur J Anaesthesiol 2015;32(11):751–8.
13. Wenzel JT, Schwenk ES, Baratta JL, et al. Managing opioid-tolerant patients in the perioperative surgical home. Anesthesiol Clin 2016;34(2):287–301.
14. Manion SC, Brennan TJ. Thoracic epidural analgesia and acute pain management. Anesthesiology 2011;115(1):181–8.
15. Nguyen LC, Sing DC, Bozic KJ. Preoperative reduction of opioid use before total joint arthroplasty. J Arthroplasty 2016;31(9 Suppl):282–7.
16. Loftus RW, Yeager MP, Clark JA, et al. Intraoperative ketamine reduces perioperative opiate consumption in opiate-dependent patients with chronic back pain undergoing back surgery. Anesthesiology 2010;113(3):639–46.
17. Kumar K, Kirksey MA, Duong S, et al. A review of opioid-sparing modalities in perioperative pain management: methods to decrease opioid use postoperatively. Anesth Analg 2017;125(5):1749–60.
18. de Klaver MJ, Buckingham MG, Rich GF. Lidocaine attenuates cytokine-induced cell injury in endothelial and vascular smooth muscle cells. Anesth Analg 2003;97(2):465–70. Table of contents.
19. Chia YY, Liu K, Wang JJ, et al. Intraoperative high dose fentanyl induces postoperative fentanyl tolerance. Can J Anaesth 1999;46(9):872–7.
20. Koppert W, Schmelz M. The impact of opioid-induced hyperalgesia for postoperative pain. Best Pract Res Clin Anaesthesiol 2007;21(1):65–83.
21. Gritsenko K, Khelemsky Y, Kaye AD, et al. Multimodal therapy in perioperative analgesia. Best Pract Res Clin Anaesthesiol 2014;28(1):59–79.
22. Hurley RW, Cohen SP, Williams KA, et al. The analgesic effects of perioperative gabapentin on postoperative pain: a meta-analysis. Reg Anesth Pain Med 2006;31(3):237–47.

23. Zhang J, Ho KY, Wang Y. Efficacy of pregabalin in acute postoperative pain: a meta-analysis. Br J Anaesth 2011;106(4):454–62.

24. Schwenk ES, Goldberg SF, Patel RD, et al. Adverse drug effects and preoperative medication factors related to perioperative low-dose ketamine infusions. Reg Anesth Pain Med 2016;41(4):482–7.

25. Deer TR, Pope JE, Hayek SM, et al. The polyanalgesic consensus conference (PACC): recommendations for intrathecal drug delivery: guidance for improving safety and mitigating risks. Neuromodulation 2017;20(2):155–76.

26. Grider JS, Brown RE, Colclough GW. Perioperative management of patients with an intrathecal drug delivery system for chronic pain. Anesth Analg 2008;107(4):1393–6.

27. Fisher R, Hassenbusch S, Krames E, et al. A consensus statement regarding the present suggested titration for prialt (ziconotide). Neuromodulation 2005;8(3):153–4.

28. Patel S, Hafez O, Sexton WJ, et al. Perioperative management of a patient with an intrathecal drug delivery device infusing ziconotide: a case report. A A Case Rep 2017;8(4):78–80.

29. Kapural L. Spinal cord stimulation for intractable chronic pain. Curr Pain Headache Rep 2014;18(4):406.

30. Mekhail NA, Cheng J, Narouze S, et al. Clinical applications of neurostimulation: forty years later. Pain Pract 2010;10(2):103–12.

31. Harrison C, Epton S, Bojanic S, et al. The efficacy and safety of dorsal root ganglion stimulation as a treatment for neuropathic pain: a literature review. Neuromodulation 2017. [Epub ahead of print].

32. Walsh KM, Machado AG, Krishnaney AA. Spinal cord stimulation: a review of the safety literature and proposal for perioperative evaluation and management. Spine J 2015;15(8):1864–9.

33. Harned ME, Gish B, Zuelzer A, et al. Anesthetic considerations and perioperative management of spinal cord stimulators: literature review and initial recommendations. Pain Physician 2017;20(4):319–29.

34. Siddiqui MA, Khan IA. Differential electrocardiographic artifact from implanted spinal cord stimulator. Int J Cardiol 2003;87(2–3):307–9.

35. Monahan K, Casavant D, Rasmussen C, et al. Combined use of a true-bipolar sensing implantable cardioverter defibrillator in a patient having a prior implantable spinal cord stimulator for intractable pain. Pacing Clin Electrophysiol 1998;21(12):2669–72.

36. Pain SA, Pain SA, Raff M, et al. Spinal cord stimulation for the management of pain: recommendations for best clinical practice. S Afr Med J 2013;103(6 Pt 2):423–30.

37. Vadivelu N, Mitra S, Kaye AD, et al. Perioperative analgesia and challenges in the drug-addicted and drug-dependent patient. Best Pract Res Clin Anaesthesiol 2014;28(1):91–101.

38. Gonzalez-Barboteo J, Porta-Sales J, Sanchez D, et al. Conversion from parenteral to oral methadone. J Pain Palliat Care Pharmacother 2008;22(3):200–5.

39. Heit HA, Gourlay DL. Buprenorphine: new tricks with an old molecule for pain management. Clin J Pain 2008;24(2):93–7.

40. Anderson TA, Quaye ANA, Ward EN, et al. To stop or not, that is the question: acute pain management for the patient on chronic buprenorphine. Anesthesiology 2017;126(6):1180–6.

41. Ohlendorf B, Grant SA. Percutaneous peripheral nerve stimulation in acute pain medicine. Curr Anesthesiol Rep 2017;7(2):220–6.

Comprehensive Acute Pain Management in the Perioperative Surgical Home

John-Paul J. Pozek, MD, Martin De Ruyter, MD,
Talal W. Khan, MD, MBA*

KEYWORDS

- Perioperative surgical home • Perioperative pain service • Chronic postsurgical pain
- Preventative analgesia • Multimodal analgesia • Opioid epidemic • Neuraxial opioids

KEY POINTS

- Establishing a perioperative surgical home (PSH) framework can lead to improved analgesic treatment of surgical patients through careful coordination of care.
- Perioperative administration of a multimodal analgesic plan, including nonopioid modalities and regional and neuraxial anesthesia techniques, can minimize postsurgical pain.
- Severe postoperative pain along with other patient- and surgery-specific factors can lead to chronic postsurgical pain.
- A preoperative assessment by a physician anesthesiologist can identify patients with behavioral risk factors for persistent postoperative opioid usage and address concerns before surgery.

INTRODUCTION

Perioperative care in the United States is plagued by fragmented care and high costs, which has spurred innovative solutions across many specialties.[1] One model is the perioperative surgical home (PSH). PSH is defined by the American Society of Anesthesiologists as "A patient-centered and physician-led multidisciplinary and team-based system of coordinated care that guides the patient throughout the entire surgical experience."[1] The Triple Aim Goals of the PSH are as follows:

1. Improve the individual experience of care
2. Improve the health of populations
3. Reduce the capita cost of care

Disclosure Statement: The authors have no relevant disclosures.
Department of Anesthesiology and Pain Medicine, University of Kansas Medical Center, 3901 Rainbow Boulevard, MS 1034, Kansas City, KS 66160, USA
* Corresponding author.
E-mail address: tkhan@kumc.edu

Anesthesiology Clin 36 (2018) 295–307
https://doi.org/10.1016/j.anclin.2018.01.007
1932-2275/18/© 2018 Elsevier Inc. All rights reserved.

Perioperative analgesia also suffers from heterogeneity of care and high costs.[2] In the current system, the surgeon is responsible for the analgesic management of most patients after they leave the postanesthesia care unit (PACU). Certain institutions have a dedicated acute pain service to treat special populations, such as opioid-tolerant patients and those receiving continuous regional or neuraxial analgesia. Within the PSH, a comprehensive perioperative analgesic plan can be coordinated before surgery with the aim of providing effective multimodal analgesia, avoiding prolonged postoperative opioid use, and mitigating the risk of transitioning from severe acute postsurgical pain to chronic postsurgical pain (CPSP).

CONSEQUENCES OF UNCONTROLLED ACUTE PAIN

Patients with uncontrolled acute pain can incur significant psychological distress, such as anxiety, depression, and impaired sleep.[3] In addition, refractory acute pain may correlate with the development of CPSP after surgery. Intense acute postsurgical pain is a risk factor across a multitude of surgeries.[4,5] Despite the reported risks associated with uncontrolled acute pain, more than 80% of patients undergoing surgery continue to report moderate to severe postsurgical pain.[5]

Although most patients will undergo surgery and return to baseline, the biopsychosocial consequences of uncontrolled acute pain are associated with dramatic economic costs. First, excessive postsurgical pain not only increases the length of hospital stay but is also one of the most common reasons for hospital readmission after discharge. In a study involving more than 20,000 patients undergoing same-day surgery, 38% of the patients who returned to the hospital reported pain as the main reason for readmission, with the average cost per patient estimated at more than $1800.[6]

Further, the development of chronic persistent pain after surgery can incur additional economic burden via lost productivity and wages in the workforce, subsequent clinic visits, and truncated reimbursement from poor patient satisfaction scores via the Hospital Consumer Assessment of Healthcare Providers and Systems survey. Pain disability that ensues as a result of CPSP has been estimated to incur the United States $43,000 annually per patient.[7] A study out of Toronto, Canada demonstrated 27% of patients reporting pain 3 months after surgery remained on opioids to manage their CPSP, thereby perpetuating the opioid epidemic.[8]

Another potential outcome of persistent pain is cognitive decline and increased risk of dementia in the elderly. A recent review of the large Health and Retirement Study database compared Americans older than 65 years who reported pain in 1998 and 2000 (labeled as persistent pain) with those who did not. After 4 biennial follow-up assessments, the group labeled *persistent pain* experienced more rapid memory loss, loss of executive functions, and an increased likelihood of developing dementia.[9]

THE ACUTE TO CHRONIC PAIN TRANSITION

Whereas many chronic pain conditions are difficult to predict because of the variability of the inciting event, CPSP is initiated after a surgical insult given a set of risk factors.[5] CPSP is pain that lasts for more than 3 to 6 months after surgery.[10] CPSP results not only in significant patient (and family) suffering and decreased quality of life but also increased health care spending and reduced functionality and work performance.[11–13] Of the many existing risk factors for CPSP, some may be modifiable and some are unmodifiable (**Table 1**). As perioperative physicians, it is imperative that we seek to identify and mitigate these risk factors throughout the perioperative continuum to reduce the development of CPSP.

Table 1	
Risk factors for developing chronic postsurgical pain	
Modifiable Risk Factors	**Nonmodifiable Risk Factors**
Preoperative pain within the site of surgery	Younger age
Severe postoperative pain	Female sex
Pain syndromes	Surgical procedure
Psychosocial factors	
Surgical approach	

Data from Pozek JP, Beausang D, Baratta JL, et al. The acute to chronic pain transition: can chronic pain be prevented? Med Clin North Am 2016;100(1):17–30; and Althaus A, Hinrichs-Rocker A, Chapman R, et al. Development of a risk index for the prediction of chronic post-surgical pain. Eur J Pain 2012;16(6):901–10.

PERSISTENT POSTSURGICAL OPIOID USE

In addition to the burden of CPSP, recent studies have shed light on persistent postsurgical opioid use. Investigators examined claims data from 36,177 adult patients with no immediate prior opioid use who underwent major or minor elective procedures between 2013 and 2014. It was noted that regardless of whether the procedure was considered major or minor, 6% of patients filled opioid prescriptions between 90 and 180 days after surgery. The investigators propose that persistent opioid use may not simply be related to whether a procedure is considered major or minor, but is more likely due to addressable patient-level predictors, including preoperative tobacco use, alcohol and substance abuse disorders, mood disorders, and preoperative pain disorders.[14] Many of these risk factors can be identified preoperatively by the physician anesthesiologist during the preoperative assessment visit. These can risk factors subsequently be addressed through either direct education interventions for tobacco cessation or partnership and consultation with psychological and psychiatric services to help reduce persistent postoperative opioid use.

IDENTIFICATION OF AT-RISK POPULATIONS

Risk factors for the acute to chronic pain transition are largely due to surgical- and patient-specific factors. Genetic and patient-related predispositions, such as young age,[4] female sex,[15] and a history of pain syndromes, such as fibromyalgia,[16] can lead to the development of chronic pain. The evidence for psychosocial factors leading to CPSP is mixed. Preoperative anxiety and depression have been identified as a risk factor for the development of CPSP after breast[15,17] and hip surgeries,[3] whereas Aasvang and colleagues[18] found that anxiety was not a factor for the development of CPSP in hernia repair. Different types of surgery have an increased incidence of CPSP **(Fig. 1)**. Although the type of surgery is an important factor, surgical technique, incision location, and surgical expertise can also influence the risk of developing CPSP.[4]

Given the wide distribution of factors, the use of one measure to predict the development of CPSP is highly unlikely.[19] Multivariate models may prove valuable in identifying risk factors. One model identified the presence of preoperative pain in the surgical field, other chronic pain, postsurgical acute pain, the presence of one or more stress symptoms, and overstraining in the 6 months before surgery as predictors for the development of CPSP with a sensitivity of 60% and a specificity of 83%.[20] All of these surgical- and patient-related risk factors must be taken into account during the patient evaluation to determine proper anesthetic and analgesic management.

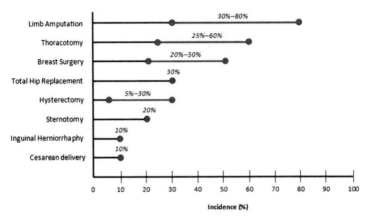

Fig. 1. Risk of developing CPSP by surgical intervention. (*Data from* Refs.[4,5,19])

PREOPERATIVE ASSESSMENT

Within the framework of the PSH, the perioperative encounter is treated as a continuum. The preoperative assessment commences soon after the decision for surgery. Anesthetic evaluation of patients should occur in a preoperative clinic, well in advance of the day of surgery, instead of occurring at the bedside minutes before the procedure. This timing allows the physician anesthesiologist ample time to perform a detailed history and physical, while coordinating further testing, treatment, prehabilitation, and optimization as indicated. Evaluation in a controlled setting can give the physician anesthesiologist necessary time to provide perioperative education, alleviate anxiety associated with the anesthetic management, and manage the patients' expectations of pain. This evaluation is instrumental to the success of the analgesic plan.[21]

Consideration of risk factors for developing CPSP is important in formulating a perioperative analgesic plan. Preexisting pain can be elucidated through the patients' history and physical. If preexisting pain is present, the physician anesthesiologist must note the pain location, pain quality, inciting factors, analgesic medications patients are taking, duration and frequency of the therapy, as well as the efficacy of any non-pharmacologic therapies or devices used by patients.

Although certain surgeries have a higher risk of developing CPSP, surgical approach can lead to persistent postsurgical pain. For example, there is a decreased incidence of chronic pain after thoracotomy with the anterolateral versus posterolateral approach.[22] Additionally, Pfannenstiel incisions demonstrate less persistent pain than midline incisions after a hysterectomy.[23] Once all factors have been reviewed, a patient- and surgery-specific analgesic plan can be formulated between the anesthetic and surgical teams. If indicated, an appropriate multimodal analgesic regimen can be initiated preoperatively.

MULTIMODAL ANALGESIA

A multimodal approach to anesthesia utilizes regional or neuraxial anesthesia and multiple different medication classes to affect different receptors with the intent of minimizing opioid consumption (**Fig. 2**). In a large review, Kehlet and colleagues[11] demonstrate positive outcomes with aggressive multimodal analgesia, with an emphasis on the completeness and appropriateness of analgesic intervention. Thus, with a mechanistic approach, different treatment options must be considered

measures to provide postoperative pain relief

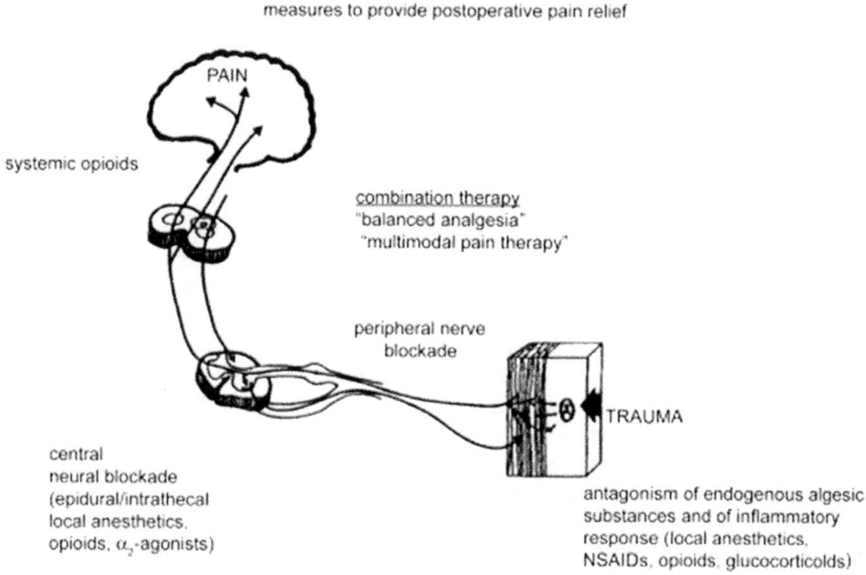

Fig. 2. Multimodal analgesic effects on the pain pathway. (*From* Kehlet H, Dahl JB. The value of "multimodal" or "balanced analgesia" in postoperative pain treatment. Anesth Analg 1993;77(5):1049; with permission.)

for different pain, such as inflammatory and neuropathic. Utilization of multimodal analgesic plans has been demonstrated to decrease opioid consumption, length of stay, and surgical complications across a wide variety of procedures, including colorectal, thoracic, and orthopedic surgery.[24–26]

Gabapentinoids act on the alpha 2-delta 2 calcium channel, reducing the hyperexcitability of dorsal horn neurons after tissue damage.[27] As part of a balanced analgesic technique, both gabapentin[28] and pregabalin[29] have shown utility in decreasing opioid consumption in large meta-analyses. Choosing the appropriate dose is important, as studies have shown that 150 mg of pregabalin 1 hour preoperatively significantly reduces opioid consumption,[30,31] whereas 50 to 75 mg preoperatively did not reduce postoperative opioids.[32]

Other medications that have shown to have benefit as part of a multimodal analgesic plan are nonsteroidal antiinflammatory drugs (NSAIDs) and acetaminophen. In a large meta-analysis by Elia and colleagues,[33] both NSAIDs and acetaminophen demonstrated opioid-sparing ability, whereas NSAIDs alone showed improved analgesia and decreased opioid-related adverse drug events. Neuraxial, truncal, and peripheral nerve blocks are an important part of a balanced anesthetic technique when feasible.

PREEMPTIVE ANALGESIA VERSUS PREVENTATIVE ANALGESIA

Controversy exists over the proper timing of analgesic therapy. In order to understand this controversy, it is important to understand the concepts of preemptive and preventative analgesia. Whereas preemptive analgesia posits that it is more important to give nociceptive treatment before surgical incision,[34] preventative analgesia encompasses all perioperative efforts to decrease pain and opioid consumption.[35] In a large review of 80 randomized controlled trials (RCTs), Møiniche and colleagues[34] demonstrated no superiority of analgesia if given before the incision.

An explanation of this phenomenon could be that tissue injury from surgical incision is not as intense, persistent, and challenging to treat as nerve injury and inflammation.[35] Thus, a perioperative analgesic regimen with a longer duration aimed at decreasing hyperalgesia and peripheral and central sensitization is more important than a solely preincisional analgesic plan.

INTRAOPERATIVE MANAGEMENT

Basic tenets for the intraoperative anesthetic plan should include multimodal techniques, optimal administration of opioids, and an anesthetic that best serves patients. This anesthetic plan includes inhalational, intravenous, or regional (peripheral or neuraxial) techniques. Although there are conflicting opinions, the choice of the anesthetic certainly may play a role in the perioperative metrics. For example, if patients receive an inhalational anesthetic and a block, they may require less opioids but may still be a risk for postoperative nausea and vomiting (PONV). If the same patients received a total intravenous anesthetic, which has been associated with less PONV, and a block, they may have a shorter, uncomplicated hospital length of stay and a more favorable impact on perioperative metrics.

The intraoperative physician anesthesiologist's focus should use techniques that provide intraoperative care with the aim that such a combination will best serve patients throughout their perioperative course. Some surgical procedures, such as those commonly associated with orthopedics, readily accommodate peripheral nerve blocks or neuraxial techniques as the intraoperative anesthetic. However, other procedures (eg, thoracotomy) typically require a general anesthetic for intraoperative care but lend themselves to regional techniques for postoperative analgesia. Used in combination, regional techniques with general anesthetics can serve the role of overall opioid reduction and extended postoperative analgesia.[21] **Table 2** lists some common surgical procedures amenable to the addition of peripheral nerve blocks as adjuvants to the overall analgesic prescription.

INTRAOPERATIVE OPIOID MINIMIZATION

Opioids are the mainstay of surgical analgesia, both intraoperatively and postoperatively. They are relatively inexpensive, titratable, readily available, and very familiar to

Table 2
Common surgical procedures and associated peripheral nerve blocks adjuvants

Surgery	Regional Techniques	
Shoulder	Interscalene	Superficial cervical plexus
Wrist	Supraclavicular/axillary	Medial, ulnar, radial nerve
Breast	PEC I and PEC II	Paravertebral
Thoracotomy[a]	PEC and serratus anterior	Intercostal
Laparotomy[a]	TAPs/rectus sheath	Quadratus lumborum
Cystectomy[a]	TAPs	Quadratus lumborum
Total hip arthroplasty[a]	Lumbar plexus	Fascia iliaca
Total knee arthroplasty	Adductor canal	Femoral nerve
Below-knee amputation[a]	Sciatic nerve	Femoral nerve
Foot/ankle	Popliteal sciatic nerve	Saphenous

Abbreviations: PEC, pectoral nerve block; TAP, transversus abdominis plane block.
[a] Epidurals are commonly used for postoperative analgesia in these procedures as well.

the health care provider. However, they are associated with numerous adverse outcomes. For today's practicing physician anesthesiologists, it is imperative that they examine their administration techniques regarding opioids and focus their attention on optimized, targeted delivery of these agents in a patient-specific manner. The overall aim is to reduce patient exposure while providing adequate analgesia, which can be achieved with a multimodal approach. Reduction of opioids accomplishes less PONV, less respiratory depression, and overall fewer perioperative complications.

In an optimized, targeted delivery, the physician anesthesiologist understands the comorbidities of their patients and weighs these complexities in determining the amount of opioids to administer to patients. Understandably, young orthopedic trauma patients may need more opioid analgesics than the elderly woman for mastectomy. Today's physician anesthesiologists should lead the movement steering away from a one-size-fits-all approach to perioperative analgesia.

INTRAOPERATIVE MULTIMODAL ANALGESIA

To accomplish these optimized goals and still meet the standard of adequate analgesia, one needs to use multimodal management. Several agents have been discussed earlier; however, *multimodal* is a broad term and encompasses approaches that include pharmacologic, nonpharmacologic, and regional block techniques. **Table 3** lists several of the pharmacologic agents that can be used intraoperatively and doses that have been reported. **Box 1** lists suggestions for nonpharmacologic approaches, which encompass categories of physical and behavioral interventions.

The role of the intraoperative anesthesia team is critical. It is the acute exposure of patients to nociceptive stimulation that they must prepare for and treat. Having a plan articulated preoperatively and understood by all participants will help guide patients through this noxious experience. It is thought that such a team-based, patient-centered approach with the emphasis on multimodal techniques will result in an optimized, targeted perioperative analgesia and overall experience.

Table 3
Multimodal agents, classification, common drugs, and dosages

Medication Class	Medication	Common Dosage
NSAIDs	Celebrex	200 mg BID
	Ketorolac	15 mg q 8 h
Acetaminophen	Tylenol	1000 mg q 8 h
Gabapentinoids	Gabapentin	300–1200 mg
	Pregabalin	75–150 mg
SNRI	Tramadol	100 mg BID
NMDA antagonists	Ketamine	Bolus: 0.5–1.0 mg/kg
		Infusion: 0.1–0.25 mg/kg/h
	Dextromethorphan	30–60 mg po BID or TID
	Magnesium	Bolus: 30–50 mg/kg
		Infusion: 10–15 mg/kg/h
Local anesthetic	Lidocaine	Bolus: 1.5 mg/kg
		Infusion: 2 mg/kg/h
Glucocorticoids	Dexamethasone	4–10 mg
Vitamin C		2 g

Abbreviations: NMDA, N-methyl-d-aspartate; SNRI, serotonin-norepinephrine reuptake inhibitor.

Box 1		
Nonpharmacologic approaches that may act as adjuvants to postoperative analgesia		
Heat	Cold/Ice	Tens
Biofeedback	Distraction	Education
Mindfulness	Coaching	Cognitive behavioral therapy

POSTOPERATIVE MANAGEMENT

As an integral part of the PSH, the physician anesthesiologist's contribution to perioperative care does not end on arrival to the PACU. Involvement can extend to resuscitation, postoperative analgesic plans, and beyond. Expert input is especially important in difficult-to-manage populations, such as opioid-tolerant patients and those with severe postsurgical pain. As discussed earlier, uncontrolled postsurgical pain can lead to deleterious physiologic changes and is a risk factor for the development of CPSP.[4]

Multiple analgesic strategies exist for the postoperative management of these patients. Severe postsurgical pain is best treated by continuing a multimodal analgesic plan consisting of regional/neuraxial analgesia, opioids, and analgesic adjuncts.

MANAGING REGIONAL ANALGESIA

Regional and neuraxial analgesia can be continued throughout the postoperative period as continuous peripheral nerve blocks (cPNBs) or continuous epidural analgesia (CEA).

There may be reticence to perform cPNBs, as they are associated with a higher cost, increased procedure time, and skill level required for adequate performance when compared with single-injection PNB (siPNBs). However, in a large meta-analysis, cPNBs demonstrated superior analgesia, decreased opioids, and increased patient satisfaction when compared with siPNBs.[36]

Another potential benefit of cPNBs is the avoidance of rebound pain that is seen after the performance of siPNBs. A meta-analysis of 23 RCTs was performed comparing pain scores and opioid usage for 48 hours after shoulder surgery with a single-injection interscalene block versus no block. Although the siPNB group had decreased pain scores up to 16 hours postoperatively and opioid consumption 12 hours postoperatively, the pain was actually greater in the siPNB group after 16 hours with a greater opioid consumption from 12 to 24 hours.[37] Similar results were seen in ankle surgery.[38] Although controlled-release local anesthetics, such as liposomal bupivacaine, offer the potential for long-acting relief through a single injection, none of these medications are currently approved for peripheral nerve blocks.

CEA can provide postoperative analgesia for a wide range of orthopedic, abdominal, and thoracic surgeries. Its use is likely to become more important, as it is included in more surgical pathways.[39] With pharmacologic and procedural expertise, the physician anesthesiologist is well suited to lead the management of CEA in the postoperative period. Important considerations in managing epidural analgesia include titrating local anesthetics, monitoring for side effects, and making the decision whether or not to include opioids in the neuraxial block (**Box 2**).

POSTOPERATIVE MULTIMODAL ANALGESIA

Extending the multimodal analgesic plan into the postoperative period has shown a benefit in pain control, but conclusive evidence on the length of time to administer medications has not been found. Acetaminophen administered in the first 24 hours

---

Box 2
Special considerations: should I use neuraxial opioids?

Neuraxial administration of opioids provides analgesia by binding opioid receptors within substantia gelatinosa. Although neuraxial opioids can have analgesic benefits, they carry side effects of pruritus, nausea, vomiting, and, the most serious, respiratory depression. The practitioner must decide if neuraxial opioids are appropriate on a case-by-case basis and after performing a history and physical. Case reports and studies with observational findings have suggested that obesity, obstructive sleep apnea, coexisting diseases, and preoperative opioid usage are associated with respiratory depression after neuraxial opioids.[45]

Timing of administration, route of administration, and type of opioid must be considered. A literature review comparing a single injection of epidural opioids with intramuscular opioids found no difference in respiratory depression, but the neuraxial group had less somnolence and sedation. The American Society of Anesthesiologists' most recent practice guideline on neuraxial opioid use found that neither epidural nor parenteral opioids were preferable for reducing the risk of respiratory depression.

The type of opioid used is important, as hydrophilic agents have an increased duration of action. The practice guideline advised against using hydrophilic neuraxial opioids in outpatient procedures. However, multiple RCTs report no difference in the frequency of respiratory depression between neuraxial administration of hydrophilic and lipophilic opioids.

---

postoperatively has been shown to reduce the morphine dose by 20%.[40] Studies of postoperative doses of gabapentinoids have ranged from a single postoperative dose to repeated doses for 30 days. Results have been mixed, but studies with the most outcomes for pain control and opioid reduction have administered doses for at least 2 weeks postoperatively.[41] Ultimately, the decision for length of postoperative analgesic regimen is patient specific, with a consideration on surgical type and after a multidisciplinary discussion with surgical and primary care teams.

PERIOPERATIVE PAIN SERVICE WITHIN THE PERIOPERATIVE SURGICAL HOME

Many institutions have an acute pain management service to manage the analgesic plan from immediately after the procedure until resumption of standard analgesic therapy. Zaccagnino and colleagues[19] proposed that the PSH allows for an expansion of the acute pain management team's role to encompass the entire perioperative episode. The team would provide proactive and continuous perioperative analgesia management after the decision is made to proceed with surgery and continue into the postdischarge phase. The focus of this team would be prevention of pain rather than reactive treatment.[19]

Multiple barriers exist to the implementation of a perioperative pain service as part of the PSH. Dissemination and implementation science has shown that implementation of a novel care team requires collaboration with a multidisciplinary team consisting of anesthesiologists, surgeons, ward nurses, and pharmacists.[42] Cooperation between these disciplines can produce pathways for care and recovery of patients at high risk for CPSP.[19]

Another important factor in the proper implementation of this team is proper education and training in perioperative analgesia. Kain and colleagues[1] suggest that to create a comprehensive PSH with integrated clinical pathways, training to incorporate the perioperative management of patients in a multiphase continuum should begin in residency. Thus, education of members would include not only perioperative analgesic management but also dissemination and implementation science, team building, and management of change.[1]

THE PERIOPERATIVE SURGICAL HOME MODEL AND ITS IMPACT ON THE OPIOID CRISIS

The recent attention to the opioid crisis in the lay media as well as scientific publications has brought about unprecedented attention to the issue of opioid prescription, use, abuse, diversion, overdose, and death. The underlying sources of the opioid crisis are multifactorial and complex. It should be recognized that the opioid crisis and the chronic pain epidemic are not one and the same but in fact overlap in significant ways. Despite opioid-related adverse effects, risks, and possible negative effects on patients and health care systems, this class of medications remains a vital analgesic option for the management of perioperative and periprocedural pain.[43]

The patient-centered, multidisciplinary, evidence-based care coordination framework of the PSH provides an ideal vehicle to help manage complex patients with chronic pain through the perioperative continuum and beyond.[44] Through preoperative patient assessment, education, and optimization, patients with chronic pain can be identified, medications and physical status optimized, and reliance on opioids possibly reduced in anticipation of surgery. Multimodal strategies can be used through intraoperative and postoperative care to minimize pain while reducing the risks associated with any analgesic class (including opioids) and analgesic interventions. Postdischarge planning, close monitoring, and coordination with a transitional pain clinic and the primary care physician should ultimately result in patients returning to baseline or better functional status and either the same or reduced opioid dose. Thus, the PSH framework has the potential to blunt the opioid crisis and improve the burden of chronic pain.

SUMMARY

A comprehensive approach to perioperative management of acute pain is important to not only reduce patient suffering and dissatisfaction but also to avoid prolonged postoperative opioid use and the development of CPSP. Implementing a PSH can streamline perioperative care. With careful coordination of care between the anesthesiology, surgery, and medicine teams, a perioperative analgesic plan can be discussed and initiated before the day of surgery and continued through recovery. Physician anesthesiologists are well suited to lead the analgesic care of surgical patients with involvement in all phases of the perioperative continuum because of expertise in acute and chronic pain management, regional anesthesia techniques, and the pharmacology of multimodal agents.

REFERENCES

1. Kain ZN, Vakharia S, Garson L, et al. The perioperative surgical home as a future perioperative practice model. Anesth Analg 2014;118:1126–30.
2. Lee A, Chan S, Chen PP, et al. Economic evaluations of acute pain service programs: a systematic review. Clin J Pain 2007;23:726–33.
3. Joshi GP, Ogunnaike BO. Consequences of inadequate postoperative pain relief and chronic persistent postoperative pain. Anesthesiol Clin North America 2005; 23:21–36.
4. Pozek JP, Beausang D, Baratta JL, et al. The acute to chronic pain transition: can chronic pain be prevented? Med Clin North Am 2016;100(1):17–30.
5. Sinatra R. Causes and consequences of inadequate management of acute pain. Pain Med 2010;11:1859–71.
6. Gan TJ, Habib AS, Miller TE, et al. Incidence, patient satisfaction, and perceptions of post-surgical pain: results from a US national survey. Curr Med Res Opin 2014;30:149–60.

7. Parsons B, Schaefer C, Mann R, et al. Economic and humanistic burden of post-trauma and post-surgical neuropathic pain among adults in the United States. J Pain Res 2013;6:459–69.

8. Huang A, Azam A, Segal S, et al. Chronic postsurgical pain and persistent opioid use following surgery: the need for a transitional pain service. Pain Manag 2016; 6(5):435–43.

9. Whitlock EL, Diaz-Ramirez LG, Glymour MM, et al. Association between persistent pain and memory decline and dementia in a longitudinal cohort of elders. JAMA Intern Med 2017;177(8):1146–53.

10. Merskey H, Bogduk N, International Association for the Study of Pain. Task force on taxonomy. Classification of chronic pain: descriptions of chronic pain syndromes and definitions of pain terms. 2nd edition. Seattle (WA): IASP Press; 1994.

11. Kehlet H, Jensen TS, Woolf CJ. Persistent postsurgical pain: risk factors and prevention. Lancet 2006;367(9522):1618–25.

12. Eriksen J, Jensen MK, Sjogren P, et al. Epidemiology of chronic non-malignant pain in Denmark. Pain 2003;106(3):221–8.

13. Stephens J, Laskin B, Pashos C, et al. The burden of acute postoperative pain and the potential role of the COX-2-specific inhibitors. Rheumatology (Oxford) 2003;42(Suppl 3):40–52.

14. Brummett CM, Waljee JF, Goesling J, et al. New persistent opioid use after minor and major surgical procedures in US adults. JAMA Surg 2017;152(6):e170504.

15. Katz J, Poleshuck EL, Andus CH, et al. Risk factors for acute pain and its persistence following breast cancer surgery. Pain 2005;199:16–25.

16. Brummett CM, Janda AM, Schueller CM, et al. Survey criteria for fibromyalgia independently predict increased postoperative opioid consumption after lower-extremity joint arthroplasty: a prospective, observational cohort study. Anesthesiology 2013;119:1434–43.

17. Tasmuth T, Estelanderb AM, Kalso E. Effect of present pain and mood on the memory of past postoperative pain in women treated surgically for breast cancer. Pain 1996;68:343–7.

18. Aasvang EK, Gmaehl E, Hansen JP, et al. Predictive risk factors for persistent postherniotomy pain. Anesthesiology 2010;112:957–69.

19. Zaccagnino MP, Badfer AM, Sang CN. The perioperative surgical home: a new role for the acute pain service. Anesth Analg 2017;125(4):1394–402.

20. Althaus A, Hinrichs-rocker A, Chapman R, et al. Development of a risk index for the prediction of chronic post-surgical pain. Eur J Pain 2012;16:901–10.

21. Wenzel JT, Schwenk ES, Baratta JL, et al. Managing opioid-tolerant patients in the perioperative surgical home. Anesthesiol Clin 2016;34(2):287–301.

22. Benedetti F, Vighetti S, Ricco C, et al. Neurophysiologic assessment of nerve impairment in posterolateral and muscle sparing thoracotomy. J Thorac Cardiovasc Surg 1998;115:841–7.

23. Brandsborg B, Nikolasjen L, Hansen CT, et al. Risk factors for chronic pain after hysterectomy: a nationwide questionnaire and database study. Anesthesiology 2007;106:1003–12.

24. Larson DW, Lovely JK, Cima RR, et al. Outcomes after implementation of a multimodal standard care pathway for laparoscopic colorectal surgery. Br J Surg 2014;101:1023–30.

25. Madani A, Fiore JF, Wang Y, et al. An enhanced recovery pathway reduced duration of stay and complications after open pulmonary lobectomy. Surgery 2015; 158:899–910.

26. Michelson JD, Addante RA, Charlson MD. Multimodal analgesia therapy reduces length of hospitalization in patients undergoing fusions of the ankle and hindfoot. Foot Ankle Int 2013;34:1526–34.

27. Gilron I. Gabapentin and pregabalin for chronic neuropathic and early postsurgical pain: current evidence and future directions. Curr Opin Anaesthesiol 2007;20:456–72.

28. Hurley RW, Cohen SP, Williams KA, et al. The analgesic effects of perioperative gabapentin on postoperative pain: a meta-analysis. Reg Anesth Pain Med 2006;31:237–47.

29. Zhang J, Ho KY, Wang Y. Efficacy of pregabalin in acute postoperative pain: a meta-analysis. Br J Anaesth 2011;106:454–62.

30. Agarwal A, Gautam S, Gupta D, et al. Evaluation of a single preoperative dose of pregabalin for attenuation of postoperative pain after laparoscopic cholecystectomy. Br J Anaesth 2008;101:700–4.

31. Balaban F, Yagar S, Özgök A, et al. A randomized, placebo-controlled study of pregabalin for postoperative pain intensity after laparoscopic cholecystectomy. J Clin Anesth 2012;24:175–8.

32. Peng PW, Li C, Farcas E, et al. Use of low-dose pregabalin in patients undergoing laparoscopic cholecystectomy. Br J Anaesth 2010;105:155–61.

33. Elia N, Lysakowski C, Tramer MR. Does multimodal analgesia with acetaminophen, nonsteroidal anti-inflammatory drugs, or selective cyclooxygenase-2 inhibitors and patient-controlled analgesia morphine offers advantages over morphine alone? Anesthesiology 2005;103:1296–304.

34. Møiniche S, Kehlet H, Dahl JB. A qualitative and quantitative systematic review of preemptive analgesia for postoperative pain relief: the role of timing of analgesia. Anesthesiology 2002;96(3):725–41.

35. Vadivelu N, Sukanya M, Schermer E, et al. Preventative analgesia for postoperative pain control: a broader concept. Local Reg Anesth 2014;7:17–22.

36. Binham AE, Fu R, Horn JL, et al. Continuous peripheral nerve block compared with single injection peripheral nerve block: a systematic review and meta-analysis of randomized controlled trials. Reg Anesth Pain Med 2012;37(6):583–94.

37. Abdallah FW, Halpern SH, Aoyama K, et al. Will the real benefits of single-shot interscalene block please stand up? A systematic review and meta-analysis. Anesth Analg 2015;120:1114–29.

38. Goldstein RY, Montero N, Jain SK, et al. Efficacy of popliteal block in postoperative pain control after ankle fracture fixation: a prospective randomized study. J Orthop Trauma 2012;26:557–61.

39. Walters TL, Mariano ER, Clark JD. Perioperative surgical home and the integral role of pain medicine. Pain Med 2015;16:1666–72.

40. Remy C, Marret E, Bonnet F. Effects of acetaminophen on morphine side effects and consumption after major surgery: meta-analysis of randomized controlled trials. Br J Anaesth 2005;94(4):505–13.

41. Schmidt PC, Ruchelli G, Mackey SC. Perioperative gabapentinoids: choice of agent, dose, timing, and effects on chronic postsurgical pain. Anesthesiology 2013;119:1215–21.

42. Colditz GA, Brownson RC, Proctor EK. The promise and challenges of dissemination and implementation research. In: Bronwon RC, Colditz GA, Proctor EK, editors. Dissemination and implementation research in health: translating science to practice. New York: Oxford University Press; 2012. p. 3–22.

43. Jahr JS, Bergese SD, Sheth KR, et al. Current perspective on the use of opioids in perioperative medicine: an evidence-based literature review, national survey of 70,000 physicians, and multidisciplinary clinical appraisal. Pain Med 2017. [Epub ahead of print].
44. Kaye AD, Helander EM, Vadivelu N, et al. Consensus statement for clinical pathway development for perioperative pain management and care transitions. Pain Ther 2017;6(2):129–41.
45. Practice guidelines for the prevention, detection, and management of respiratory depression associated with neuraxial opioid administration: an updated report by the American Society of Anesthesiologists Task Force on neuraxial opioids and the American Society of Regional Anesthesia and Pain Medicine. Anesthesiology 2016;124:535–52.

Anesthesiology's Future with Specialists in Population Health

Mike Schweitzer, MD, MBA*

KEYWORDS

- Population health medicine • Population health management
- Anesthesiologists or specialists in population health • Specialists in ACO
- Anesthesiologists in ACO • Specialists in CIN
- Anesthesiologists in value-based care • Specialists in value-based care

KEY POINTS

- Engaging anesthesiologists and other specialists in population health medicine in an Accountable Care Organizations (ACOs) or Clinically Integrated Networks (CINs) improves the Triple Aim.
- Organization of specialty practices into the population health delivery system requires a change in culture, transparency in key metrics, focused action plans, and effective care management processes.
- In population health medicine, often it is not primary care, but rather the specialists' care teams, that are responsible for most of the overall spending for health care.
- Patient-centric care is often characterized by patients sitting on committees of the population health organization to represent their unique perspective and needs.
- Specialists should engage in "shadow bundles" to improve quality and reduce costs under the egis of an ACO or CIN instead of through a direct payer contract.

INTRODUCTION

There are many evolving definitions and concepts for the term "Population Health." In 2003, Dr David Kindig proposed a definition in the *American Journal of Public Health* as "the health outcomes of a group of individuals, including the distribution of such outcomes within the group."[1] Kindig and Stoddart argued that the field of population health included health outcomes, patterns of health determinants, and policies and interventions that link these 2. In 2015, Dr Kindig[2] agreed with a further clarification of

Disclosure Statement: Employee of Premier Inc and Chief Clinical Officer for American Society of Anesthesiologists' Perioperative Surgical Home Learning Collaborative.
Population Health, Premier Inc, PSH Learning Collaborative, Clearwater, FL, USA
* 2672 3rd Avenue South, Clearwater, FL 33759.
E-mail address: mkschweitzer1@gmail.com

Anesthesiology Clin 36 (2018) 309–320
https://doi.org/10.1016/j.anclin.2018.01.008
1932-2275/18/© 2018 Elsevier Inc. All rights reserved.

anesthesiology.theclinics.com

"Population Health Medicine" as "the iterative process of strategically and proactively managing clinical and financial opportunities to improve health outcomes and patient engagement, while also reducing costs." This latter definition can be more easily applied to a population of patients with perioperative care or periprocedural care. This definition of Population Health Medicine focuses on the clinical opportunities that may include health care determinates of health, such as social and physical conditions of the environment where people live.

Although the title of this article is focused on anesthesiologists, the reality is that the future of anesthesia in population health medicine is closely linked to the future of surgeons and other medical specialists. This article seeks to align closely the strategies and tactics of specialists caring for populations of patients in population health medicine alternative value-based payment models such as Accountable Care Organizations (ACOs), Clinically Integrated Networks (CINs), and bundled payments.[3] The Perioperative Surgical Home (PSH) and Enhanced Recovery After Surgery models specifically seek to transform perioperative care through achieving the Institute for Healthcare Improvement Triple Aim of improving the health of the surgical population. The success of the PSH model is largely predicated on anesthesiologists, surgeons, and other clinicians understanding and applying the principles of population health medicine.[4] Specialists have roles in population health medicine coordination of care with diagnosis and treatment, transitions across settings, reducing avoidable emergency department (ED) visits and hospitalizations, and in multispecialty complex patient management. For inpatients, specialists can concentrate on hospital throughput, minimizing avoidable adverse events and readmissions, early mobility, pain management, and performance improvements. Specialists who are only intent on preserving volume at the expense of best practices have no role in population health medicine.

HEALTH POLICY ACCELERATING SHIFT TO POPULATION HEALTH

The US health care system is undergoing a transformation as government and commercial health insurers shift from paying based on volume to paying based on the value of services health providers deliver. Much of the history of physicians in population health and population health medicine has been focused on primary care physicians. The creation of the attribution rules for the Centers for Medicare and Medicaid Services (CMS) ACOs in 2010 was heavily slanted to favor primary care physicians as the drivers. In 2017, the Quality Payment Program (QPP) under the Medicare Access and CHIP Reauthorization Act (MACRA) law, the current 31 metrics for both ACOs and the subset of 15 metrics reported for the Merit-Based Incentive Payment System (MIPS) are still essentially primary care–oriented measures. As a result, often any savings in ACOs are distributed predominantly to primary care physicians. This shared savings distribution will be discussed in more detail later. The main point is that the future of anesthesiologists in population health medicine is closely aligned with other specialists working together to demonstrate their value.

The nationwide growth in ACOs and other Alternative Payment Models (APMs), such as bundled payment models, has accelerated support for value-based care. Today there are more than 900 active public and private ACOs in the United States, covering more than 32 million people. This amount will grow in January 2018 with the new CMS ACOs beginning. Although Medicare contracts exemplify about 30% of the covered lives in ACOs, commercial contracts embody nearly 60% and Medicaid covers about another 12%.[5]

APMs are seeing significant success, because Medicare ACOs have documented a savings of approximately $2 billion and reported measureable improvements in quality.

All of the Next Gen and Pioneer ACOs in Premier's Advanced Population Health Management Collaborative achieved shared savings in 2016. For example, Pioneer ACO Banner Health in Phoenix's net savings was $15.4 million with their 42,000 attributed lives ($365 per beneficiary) and Next Gen ACO Triad Health Network/Cone Health of Greensboro, North Carolina net savings was $11 million with their 27,800 covered lives ($394 per beneficiary).[6] The MACRA, which was passed by a Republican Congress in 2015, also creates positive incentives for clinicians to move away from fee for service in favor of APMs through the QPP.

POPULATION HEALTH MANAGEMENT ORGANIZATION FRAMEWORK

To be most effective as a specialist involved in Population Health Medicine, one must first understand the Population Health Management Organization (PHMO) framework that organizes the management of a population of patients. Many organizations first began to embrace this framework (**Fig. 1**) or a similar framework in 2010 after the enactment of the Affordable Care Act. Implementation of contemporary governance and operational strategies and tactics to align providers and payers to manage a population is a major paradigm shift. Collaborating as partners, this multitude of entities requires a blueprint to establish deeper and broader interactions based on transparency, shared value plans, and joint management of population health. ACOs are groups of doctors, hospitals, and other health care providers, who come together voluntarily to give coordinated high-quality care to their patients. The stated goal of CMS is for traditional fee-for-service Medicare payments shifting to APM by 50% in 2018.[3]

At the center of this framework is the population the ACO is managing. The foundation to coordinate the health of these people is the close interactions of the primary care providers in a patient-centered medical home (PCMH) and a high-value network (HVN) of key specialists. Surrounding and supporting the PCMH and HVN is a medical neighborhood of providers, including pharmacists/pharmacy, behavioral health, ancillary providers, long-term care facilities, public health agencies, palliative/hospice care,

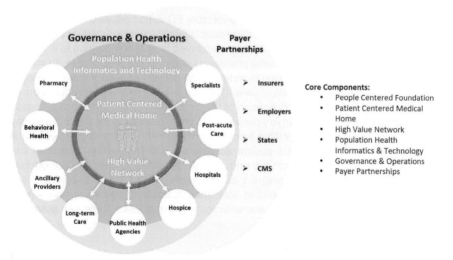

Fig. 1. Premier ACO model for population health management. (*Courtesy of* Premier, Inc, Washington, DC.)

hospitals, postacute care (PAC), and other supporting specialists. All of these are linked closely by population health informatics and technology (PHIT). The outer ring of these concentric circles is governance and operations. Aligned in another circle that overlaps in a Venn diagram are payer partnerships with insurers, employers, states, and CMS. The lesson that more than 70 organizations have learned in the Premier Collaboratives is the crucial need for providers to build effective fundamental capabilities, gain experience, and achieve success with a 1-sided risk APM model before pursuing and engaging in a 2-sided risk model with a government or commercial payer.[7]

People are at the center of this model. Patients often sit on committees of the population health organization to represent their unique perspective and needs.

However, people-centered care requires more than coordination across the continuum of care; careful attention must be directed to the entire experience at every place and person at which they interact with the ACO. Patients and clinicians must have easy access to medical records to eliminate the constant repetitive questions about their basic medical history. This access to the universal medical record is critical to transitions of care to ensure a consistent care plan and communication at the appropriate level of literacy. The population health leaders in each community must monitor individual's experiences and be prepared to address any identified issues. Other considerations include methods to enhance patient education and access to care. It is important to implement protocols and processes to help patients get the right care at the right place and time, taking into consideration specific patient needs.

The transition to value-based care in a population health management framework places a great emphasis on the need to transition primary care practices to APM like PCMHs. This transition requires a commitment for a journey to a new focus on the health of their population rather than only treating illness. There must be network-wide capability to deliver comprehensive, high-value primary care services that meets the CMS triple aim for "Better Care, Smarter Spending, and Healthier People."[8]

The HVN aligns key specialists in a medical neighborhood to manage a population across the continuum. A narrow network of engaged and committed specialists can deliver high value by optimizing the medical conditions of the moderate- to high-risk patients and reducing complications and avoidable ED visits/hospitalizations. Often anesthesiologists and many surgical/medical specialties are not included in an organization such as an ACO or CIN because of the perceived lack of contribution to high-value care. Nevertheless, engaged specialty physician leaders can work closely with an interdisciplinary team of providers willing to redesign the delivery of perioperative or periprocedural care for the entire episode of care. This care delivery redesign may start from the decision for an intervention, optimization of the patient's medical conditions before the procedure, in the hospital or surgery center, and extend beyond to the first 30 to 90 days after discharge. Engaged specialist leaders consequently provide high-quality cost-effective care with exceptional patient experience. Re-engineering speciality care necessitates working closely with the primary care providers to identify the moderate- to high-risk patients and focusing on individualizing their care in a common care pathway. It is essential for the HVN to have the capability to deliver comprehensive, high-value specialty and ancillary care services that meets CMS Triple Aim goals.

RISK-STRATIFIED CARE MANAGEMENT

One key to Population Health Medicine is a systematic risk stratification of individual patients and managing each category as a specific segment of the population. This care can be managed in a medical neighborhood that may include a PCMH, oncology home, PSH, or other providers working together to provide highly reliable care. A transitional care clinic or perioperative care clinic dedicated to managing the higher-risk patients in the weeks before and after surgery or a procedure is an effective population health medicine tactic.[9] Care management is the set of services intended to improve the health of patients, especially those with complex health care needs. These services include those provided by a perioperative or periprocedural care team that reaches out to patients and works with them to understand their health needs and to coordinate care across the medical neighborhood.

The goal of risk-stratified care management is to manage each segment of this risk pyramid differently (**Fig. 2**). At the base of the pyramid, the largest segment of the population is the well or healthy patients. The goal with this lowest-risk population is to keep people healthy and avoid individuals moving up the risk pyramid. The second lowest section of the risk pyramid is the rising-risk patients, who need education and activation to prevent further disease development. The focus is on prevention and education. Care coordination for the moderate-risk segment of the pyramid adds in medication management and therapy adherence support. It is important to monitor the care team's performance by tracking patient data and comparing it with national guidelines or internal benchmarks. The care team provides education to prevent increase in the severity of each chronic disease and the increase in the number of chronic diseases experienced by each individual. The moderate- to high-risk patients involve a proactive, team-based approach to care that focuses on prevention, early intervention, and close partnerships with patients and their families to tightly manage chronic conditions.

POPULATION HEALTH PERIOPERATIVE/PERIPROCEDURAL RISK PYRAMID

The high-risk patients often have 4 or more chronic diseases or chronic diseases at a more advanced stage. These patients often have specific care managers dedicated to

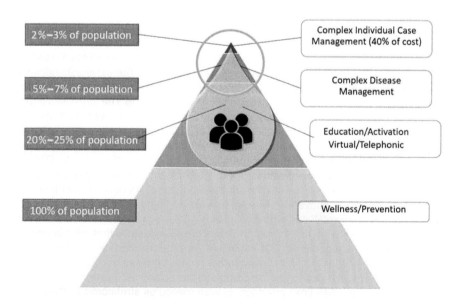

Fig. 2. Population health perioperative/periprocedural risk pyramid.

managing their care and educating the patients and families. The care team provides patient self-management support. Proactive approaches include assuring the patients have regular clinic visits to assure compliance, monitoring patient progress/laboratory tests, identifying appropriate care plans, and recommending changes to care plans by including prompts in the patient's personal electronic health record. The 2% to 3% of highest-risk patients often represent 40% to 50% of the total cost of care for a specific patient population in an accountable care organization or acute care episode.

A Health Affairs Study in April 2017 highlighted that the ACO beneficiaries who were in the top 5% of Medicare spending had an annual spend of greater than $81,461.[10] Complications after surgery necessitating ED visits and readmissions are prime candidates for being in the top 5%. This critical 90-day perioperative period can push these higher-risk patients toward the top 5% spend for the entire year. A study in 2009 demonstrated that the baseline cost of isolated coronary artery bypass grafting (CABG) cases with no complications was $26,056. Increases in costs because of complications for isolated CABG patients were greatest for those cases involving prolonged ventilation ($40,704), renal failure ($49,128), mediastinitis ($62,773), and operative mortality ($49,242) beyond the base cost for CABG surgery.[11]

Another study highlighted the high cost of complications for total hip arthroplasty (THA) or total knee arthroplasty (TKA). Surgical complications accounted for 54% of the THA readmissions and 44% of the TKA readmissions. The increase in costs over the baseline cost for surgery without complications was $36,038 for THA and $38,953 for TKA.[12]

One cost study on lumbar spinal fusion for spinal stenosis and spondylolisthesis with posterolateral spinal fusion illustrated that mean costs per case were $27,946. However, the average Medicare payment was $36,230 ± $17,020, $46,840 ± $31,350, and $61,610 ± $46,580 at 3 months, 1 year, and 2 years after surgery, respectively.[13] All these examples of increased costs for complications are extremely important when an organization is responsible for the total cost of care annually for a population. As noted previously, a savings of a couple hundred dollars per patient can generate huge overall savings for an ACO. Coordinated perioperative care provides a significant opportunity for improved quality and decreased costs.

PREOPTIMIZATION PHASE

The preoptimization phase begins with patient and family engagement/activation to become an integral part of their success in the acute care episode. There is an initial assessment and triage as necessary. Many common protocols include identification and managing preoperative anemia or nutritional deficiencies, diabetes protocol for those with a high HgA$_{1c}$, body mass index protocol, physical therapy assessment/education, and smoking cessation. Risk tools can be used to assess the risk of postprocedure skilled nursing facility (SNF) utilization. Advanced practice practitioners (APPs) as well as social workers and care managers under the direction of the perioperative care team are indispensable. Patient/family education and appropriate setting of expectations are part of the preoptimization phase. Finally, the transitional care plan for admission, surgery/procedure, immediate after recovery, and long-term recovery phases are outlined and agreed upon.

For those specialists affiliated with a Medicare ACO, such as the Medicare Shared Savings Program (MSSP) Track 1 program, there are 15 measures that are a subset of the 31 MSSP ACO measures in 2017 that are reported as part of the APM-MIPS scoring (**Table 1** lists the 31 MSSP measures).[14] The diabetes composite measure has 2 submeasures and both must be completed to qualify. All these measures are reported through the CMS Web Interface. Eleven measures are scored as they have available benchmarks (1 of the 11 measures is the diabetes composite measure,

Table 1
2017 31 Medicare Shared Savings Program measures

ACO Measure No.	Measure Title	NQF No.	Measure Steward	Method of Data Submission
Domain: care coordination/patient safety				
ACO-8	Risk-Standardized, All Condition Readmission	1789 (adapted)	CMS	Claims
ACO-35	Skilled Nursing Facility 30-day All-Cause Readmission Measures	2510 (adapted)	CMS	Claims
ACO-36	All-Cause Unplanned Admissions for Patients with Diabetes	N/A[a]	CMS	Claims
ACO-37	All-Cause Unplanned Admissions for Patients with Heart Failure	N/A	CMS	Claims
ACO-38	All-Cause Unplanned Admissions for Patients with Multiple Chronic Conditions	N/A	CMS	Claims
ACO-43	Acute Composite (AHRQ Prevention Quality Indicator #91)	N/A	AHRQ	Claims
ACO-11	Use of Certified EHR Technology	N/A	CMS	QPP data
ACO-12	Medication Reconciliation Post Discharge	97	NCQA[b]	Web interface
AC0-13	Falls: Screening for Future Fall Risk	101	AMA/PCPI/NCQA	Web interface
ACO-44	Use of Imaging Studies for Low Back Pain	52	NCQA	Claims
Domain: Preventive Health				
ACO-14	Preventive Care and Screening: Influenza Immunization	41	AMA/PCPI[c]	Web interface
ACO-15	Pneumonia Vaccination Status for Older Adults	43	NCQA	Web interface
ACO-16	Preventive Care and Screening: Body Mass Index Screening and Follow-Up	421	CMS	Web interface
ACO-17	Preventive Care and Screening: Tobacco Use: Screening and Cessation Intervention	28	AMA/PCPI	Web interface
ACO-18	Preventive Care and Screening: Screening for Clinical Depression and Follow-up Plan	418	CMS	Web interface
ACO-19	Colorectal Cancer Screening	34	NCQA	Web interface
ACO-20	Breast Cancer Screening	N/A	NCQA	Web interface
ACO-42	Statin Therapy for the Prevention and Treatment of Cardiovascular Disease	N/A	N/A	Web interface
Domain: at-risk population				
Depression				
ACO-40	Depression Remission at 12 Months	710	MNCM	Web interface

(continued on next page)

Table 1 (continued)				
ACO Measure No.	**Measure Title**	**NQF No.**	**Measure Steward**	**Method of Data Submission**
Diabetes				
ACO-27	Diabetes: Hemoglobin A1c Poor Control	59	NCQA	Web interface
ACO-41	Diabetes: Eye Exam	55	NCQA	Web interface
Hypertension				
ACO-28	Controlling High Blood Pressure	18	NCQA	Web interface
IVD				
ACO-30	Ischemic Vascular Disease (IVD): use of Aspirin or Another Antithrombotic	68	NCQA	Web interface

[a] National Committee for Quality Assurance (NCQA).
[b] American Medical Association (AMA), PCPI® (see http://www.thepcpi.org/).
[c] Not applicable (N/A).
Adapted from RTI International. Accountable Care Organization. Quality measure narrative specifications. 2017. Available at: https://www.cms.gov/Medicare/Medicare-Fee-for-Service-Payment/sharedsavingsprogram/Downloads/2017-Reporting-Year-Narrative-Specifications.pdf. Accessed January 22, 2018; with permission.

which has 2 metrics A1c poor control and diabetes-related eye examination). Three measures are not scored, because there are no existing benchmarks (medicine reconciliation after discharge, depression remission, and statin therapy).

Initially specialists often think that the ACO 31 measures and the 15 APM-MIPS measures are predominately primary care measures. However, when specialists approach episodic care in a team-based interdisciplinary approach, the care redesign can include most if not all of these ACO and APM-MIPS measures. The depression and diabetes composite measures often have the most struggle for completion and monitoring. Many of the other measures can be achieved and reported by nonphysicians.

ALTERNATIVE PAYMENT MODELS-MERIT-BASED INCENTIVE PAYMENT SYSTEM QUALITY REPORTING

The ACO has 2 separate reporting requirements. The first are the 31 measures for the ACO quality score. The second is the APM-MIPS reporting for the eligible clinicians that are identified providers in the ACO (**Box 1**).

Collecting and reporting many of the 31 measures (including the APM-MIPS subset of measures) for those moderate- to high-risk patients that are managed perioperatively will demonstrate value for the ACO. By contributing to improving the ACO quality scores in addition to reducing complications, the specialists on the perioperative team have a valid claim to share in any savings generated. Anesthesiologists and other specialists do not need to be personally collecting many of these metrics but can be leaders on the team that has accountability for collecting these metrics.

INTRAOPERATIVE OR PROCEDURE PHASE

Specialists responsible for the phase that is associated with the intraoperative or procedure must assure that the correct personnel for patient acuity and surgery are available, for example, "right person, right time, right place, all the time." Multimodal

---

Box 1
Medicare Shared Savings Program Quality Payment Program subset of Accountable Care Organizations measures

Fall Risk Screening (CARE-2/ACO 13)

DM Composite
- HbA1c Poor Control (DM-2/ACO 27)
- Eye Examination (DM-7/ACO 41)

Controlling High BP (HTN-2/ACO 28)

IVD & Use of Aspirin (IVD-2/ACO 30)

Breast CA Screening (PREV-5/ACO 20)

Colorectal CA Screening (PREV-6/ACO 19)

Flu Immunization (PREV-7/ACO 14)

Pneumonia Vaccination (PREV-8/ACO 15)

BMI Screening & F/u (PREV-9/ACO 16)

Tobacco Screening/Cessation (PREV-10/ACO 17)

Depression Screening and F/u (PREV-12/ACO 18)

Depression Remission (MH-1/ACO 40)

Statin Therapy (PREV-13/ACO 42)

Med Rec Post Discharge (CARE-1/ACO 12)

Fifteen quality measures for the reporting for eligible clinicians in the MSSP Track 1 ACO.

---

analgesia, deep vein thrombosis/antibiotic prophylaxis, carbohydrate loading, normothermia, avoidance of salt and water overload, and appropriate short-acting anesthesia, including possible regional blocks and postoperative nausea or vomiting (PONV), should all be addressed and protocols developed and adopted. Attention is given to reducing variation and adopting leading practices.

Working with the value analysis team for product and supply standardization based on the best available evidence is a leading practice. Strategic collaboration with vendors for patient outcomes-based negotiations and pricing agreements based on savings/revenue arising from quality is a great tactic. New product or technology requests should be evaluated for approval or denial based on evidence. Approvals may be unrestricted or restricted by appropriate criteria such as place, patient, proficiency, and pathology.

IMMEDIATE POSTOPERATIVE PHASE

The immediate postoperative phase has several key components starting with prevention of PONV and pain control to permit early ambulation. Early oral nutrition, early removal of a Foley catheter (if present), and reinforcing appropriate expectations for time of discharge and postdischarge location/care. Throughout the different perioperative/periprocedural transitions, consistent handovers and communications of the care plan for each patient must be standardized.

LONG-TERM RECOVERY PHASE

The long-term recovery phase begins at discharge. However, the planning and education begin soon after the decision for surgery or a procedure is made. Moderate- to high-risk patients that were managed preadmission must already have a plan for their care before discharge. If the primary care providers cannot support access to care in the first 2 to 10 days, then consider expanding your preoperative care clinic to a transitional care clinic to manage the moderate- to high-risk patients in the first few weeks after discharge. Care navigators and APPs can be critical team members to monitor and identify early issues with the moderate- to high-risk patients. Special attention should be directed at the Agency for Healthcare Research and Quality (AHRQ)-identified ambulatory-sensitive conditions, such as diabetes, congestive heart failure, chronic obstructive pulmonary disease, hypertension, pneumonia, dehydration, and urinary tract infections, to avoid unnecessary ED visits or readmissions.

POSTACUTE CARE NETWORK DEVELOPMENT

When narrowing your network, it is critical to know the capabilities of each facility that you work with and use correct placement for patients. Your perioperative team should be aware of the quality ratings, readmission rates, patient satisfaction scores, and average length of stay by diagnosis of network facilities. When codeveloping care pathways and education, your team should create cross-continuum care pathways and engage in education to maintain seamless, integrated care for patients. Standardization of processes across the continuum is also key to this step. Integrate current bundles initiatives with PAC network development efforts. Establish communication links between each SNF and each PCMH practice to ensure continuity of care. Consider on-site nurse practitioners or physician assistants to work with selected medical directors to make daily rounds on high-risk patients. Finally, you should partner with postacute facilities on readmission avoidance programs by deploying clear protocols and expectations. When partnering for readmission avoidance, root-cause analyses must be used for all readmission challenges, and your team should collaborate on quality-improvement strategies to correct problems. Develop dashboards for each SNF to track and trend performance and provide routine feedback.

PALLIATIVE CARE AND END OF LIFE

- Reduce delays of palliative/hospice care for a patient with serious illness who has physical, psychological, social, or spiritual distress because they are pursuing disease-directed treatment.
- Incorporate palliative care programs and training for acute and ambulatory settings.
- Assess use of advanced directives at a practice level and market level using the electronic medical records data.
- Establish palliative care outpatient and inpatient services, if not already implemented in your community.
- Engage local community resources to increase awareness and acceptance of end-of-life discussions before they become urgent.

Monitor use of hospice days and palliative care consults to assess use by patients and their families.

POPULATION HEALTH INFORMATICS AND TECHNOLOGY

It is important to integrate the PHIT strategy, planning, and resources with the existing health care organizations in the community. Coordinating information capture, documentation, and sharing of information across all providers is important. Many organizations are optimizing patient and provider engagement and care management through technology and informatics. It is obligatory to have true health information exchange and electronic health records connectivity between physician, hospital, and PAC providers. PHIT must provide timely, accurate, actionable, and comparable data to the PHMO, physicians, clinicians, and PAC providers.

GOVERNANCE AND OPERATIONS

Best practice is a physician-led PHMO governance structure. A wide variety of physician representatives from primary care, specialty care, and geography, who have demonstrated leadership and influence capabilities are crucial. Effective and passionate physician leaders who can influence colleagues are critical to implement focused action plans to improve key performance metrics. Professional management in a dyad structure enhances performance and growth. Communication, engagement strategies, and financial management are all essential to success. The dyad leadership must align physician incentive payment/compensation structures.

PAYER PARTNERSHIPS

First assess payer partners in your region to identify those who are interested in or have experience in value-based payment models. Then establish or reshape your relationships with those identified payer partners. Collaborate with these payers to manage population experience. Coordinate and optimize performance under QPP to leverage both CMS and commercial payers. In addition, some ACOs are engaging specialist teams in "shadow bundles" to improve quality and reduce costs for their attributed population. "Shadow bundles" take advantage of the concepts discussed in Drs Stanley W. Stead and Sharon K. Merrick's article, "Bundled Payments and Hidden Costs," in this issue but are managed under the umbrella of an ACO or CIN instead of through a direct payer contract.

Keys to success from the perspective of major health plans are as follows:

- Provide actionable and comparable data to physicians
- Focused action plans in key performance improvement areas
- Effective care management processes
- Network of high-value PAC providers
- Effective and passionate physician leaders with aligned physician incentive payment/compensation structures
- Increased capture of utilization in network (market share growth)
- Complete and accurate coding for risk acuity adjustment
- Work with providers with a Medicare ACO to have a complementary Medicare Advantage as well as commercial program/contract

SUMMARY

Many lessons can be learned from the more than 900 organizations that are participating in population health management nationwide. When evaluating the CMS goals of "Better Care, Smarter Spending, and Healthier People" in population health medicine, it is often not the care provided by primary care teams that increase the costs, but rather the specialty care teams that are the highest proportion of the overall spend for health care. Engaging specialists in an ACO or CIN in population health medicine is a prerequisite to be successful in improving the quality of care by reducing complications, unnecessary utilization, avoidable ED visits/readmissions, and total cost of care. In addition, some ACOs are engaging specialist teams in "shadow bundles" to improve quality and reduce costs for their attributed population. Creating patient-centric, physician-lead, interdisciplinary care teams to redesign the delivery of care across the continuum of the episode of care is a successful approach for commercial or CMS value-based payments.

REFERENCES

1. Kindig D, Stoddart G. What is population health? Am J Public Health 2003;93: 380–3.
2. Kindig DA. What are we talking about when we talk about population health? In Health Affairs Blog. 2015. Available at: http://healthaffairs.org/blog/2015/04/06/what-are-we-talking-about-when-we-talk-about-population-health/. Accessed October 20, 2017.
3. Schweitzer M, Vetter T. The perioperative surgical home: more than smoke and mirrors? Anesth Analg 2016;123:524–8.
4. Boudreaux AM, Vetter TR. A primer on population health management and its perioperative application. Anesth Analg 2016;123:63–70.
5. Muhlestein D, Saunders R, McClellan M. Growth of ACOs and alternative payment models in 2017. Health Aff 2017. Available at: http://www.healthaffairs.org/do/10.1377/hblog20170628.060719/full/. Accessed October 25, 2017.
6. CMS.gov. Shared savings program Accountable Care Organizations (ACO) PUF. Available at: https://www.cms.gov/Research-Statistics-Data-and-Systems/Downloadable-Public-Use-Files/SSPACO/. Accessed October 31, 2017.
7. Damore J, Hardaway B. Ready, risk, reward: building successful two-sided risk models. 2017. Available at: https://www.premierinc.com/. Accessed November 1, 2017.
8. Burwell S. Better care. Smarter spending. Healthier people: paying providers for value, not volume. 2015. Available at: https://www.cms.gov/Newsroom/Media ReleaseDatabase/Fact-sheets/2015-Fact-sheets-items/2015-01-26-3.html. Accessed October 20, 2017.
9. Sibert K, Schweitzer MI. Practice anesthesiology - what could population health possibly have to do with me? ASA Monitor 2017;81(7):40–2.
10. Hsu J, Vogeli C, Price M, et al. Substantial physician turnover and beneficiary 'churn' in a large medicare pioneer ACO. Health Aff (Millwood) 2017;36(4):640–8.
11. Speir A, Kasirajan V, Barnett SD, et al. Additive costs of postoperative complications for isolated coronary artery bypass grafting patients in Virginia. Ann Thorac Surg 2009;88:40–5 [discussion: 45–6].
12. Clair AJ, Evangelista PJ, Lajam CM, et al. Cost analysis of total joint arthroplasty readmissions in a bundled payment care improvement initiative. J Arthroplasty 2016;31(9):162–1865.
13. Ong K, Auerbach J, Lau E, et al. Perioperative outcomes, complications, and costs associated with lumbar spinal fusion in older patients with spinal stenosis and spondylolisthesis. Neurosurg Focus 2014;36(6):E5.
14. CMS.gov. Accountable Care Organization 2017 Quality Measure Narrative Specifications. 2017. Available at: https://www.cms.gov/Medicare/Medicare-Fee-for-Service-Payment/sharedsavingsprogram/Downloads/2017-Reporting-Year-Narrative-Specifications.pdf. Accessed October 28, 2017.

Integrating Academic and Private Practices

Challenges and Opportunities

Aviva Regev, MD, MBA[a], Aman Mahajan, MD, PhD, MBA[b],*

KEYWORDS

- Academic medical center • Merger • Consolidation • Organizational culture
- Academic anesthesiology • Private practice anesthesiology
- Future models of anesthesia

KEY POINTS

- Academic medical centers' model of high-acuity, high-cost care with clinical revenues cross-subsidizing research and education is at risk in the current landscape of health care reform.
- Consolidation of academic and community medical centers through mergers or partnerships provides one mechanism to diversify, increase regional presence, and achieve economies of scale.
- Culture clash between organizations is a major but often ignored factor in failure to achieve a merger's full potential and may even contribute to complete dissolution.
- A merger of academic and private practice anesthesiology groups can benefit both, but cultural differences are likely to play a major role in successful consolidation.

INTRODUCTION

Health care, like any industry, is not immune to market pressures. As payment models and care delivery systems are increasingly pushed toward improving efficiency and value, providers and hospitals must respond, and academic medical centers (AMCs) are no exception. AMCs have historically been relatively protected from competitive forces owing to their large size, reputation, and multiple revenue sources. In the current landscape, however, even these ivory towers have been impacted by the forces affecting the market as a whole. One avenue that some centers are pursuing to enhance their competitive advantage is through mergers or partnerships with community health systems.

Conflicts of Interest: None.
[a] Department of Anesthesiology and Perioperative Medicine, UCLA Health, 757 Westwood Plaza, Suite 3325, Los Angeles, CA 90095-7403, USA; [b] Department of Anesthesiology and Perioperative Medicine, UCLA Health, 757 Westwood Plaza, Suite 2331-L, Los Angeles, CA 90095-7403, USA
* Corresponding author.
E-mail address: amahajan@mednet.ucla.edu

Anesthesiology Clin 36 (2018) 321–332
https://doi.org/10.1016/j.anclin.2018.01.012
1932-2275/18/© 2018 Elsevier Inc. All rights reserved.

DIFFERENTIATING THE ACADEMIC MEDICAL CENTERS

AMCs are defined by their tripartite mission of patient care, research, and education (**Fig. 1**). The interplay of research, education, and advanced care improves each mission separately and collectively. They are typically affiliated with a medical school as well as other health care professional schools, laboratory facilities, and programs for research from bench to bedside, large faculty practice groups, and residency training programs. They tend to enjoy strong name recognition and reputation, and are known for pioneering advancements in medical care. Although only 6% of the nation's hospitals are AMCs, they provide 20% of the hospital care in the country and receive more than 40% of patients who are transferred from community hospitals for higher level of care.[1] Compared with community hospitals, AMCs tend to care for high-risk, higher complexity patients, and provide a highly disproportionate share of intensive and specialized services, including 50% of solid organ transplants, 61% of level 1 regional trauma centers, 62% of pediatric intensive care units, and 75% of burn care units.[1] Besides the differences in the patient care, there are other significant differences in local practices and culture between the AMCs and private practices (**Box 1**).

Traditional Academic Medical Center Revenue Streams

AMCs have traditionally benefited from a combination of revenue streams. The bulk of this comes from payment for clinical services, including Medicare, Medicaid, and private insurance reimbursements, copayments, and self-payments, and comprises 85% of annual revenues. Research grants and contracts account for 12% of AMCs revenue, with federal funding the largest source, followed by industry and nonprofit foundations. The remaining 3% of AMC revenue comes from tuition, gifts, and endowments.[2] AMCs receive nearly $10 billion in annual funding from Medicare for direct and indirect graduate medical education, as well as $3.9 billion from Medicaid and $1.4 from the Veteran's health Adminitration.[3] Revenues are then distributed across the 3 missions, resulting in cross-funding of research and education from clinical revenues (**Fig. 2**).

Financial Implications

Providing high-acuity, highly specialized care while cross-subsidizing research and educational missions drives the cost structure of AMCs higher than that of non-AMCs. Other factors, including greater investment in clinical information technology

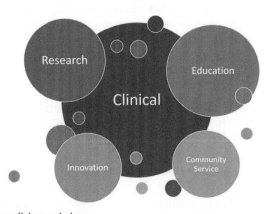

Fig. 1. Academic medicine: missions.

Box 1
Differences between AMCs and private practice models

Academic Medical Center	Private Practice
1 Tertiary/quaternary care of patients for advanced or experimental therapies in multidisciplinary teams	Flexibility in clinical practice pattern/style with lesser acuity and complexity of patient care
2 Opportunities for investigative original research/trials; expectation of scholarly academic productivity	Near 100% clinical practice with no expectations to participate in research or scholarly work
3 Participation in education and training of medical students, residents and fellows	Interest in business aspects of the private practice and efficient health care delivery
4 Nonsalary benefits (dedicated academic/nonclinical time; funded professional travel and education; discounted college tuition rates for children of faculty)	Greater salary compensation; ability to form individual corporations
5 Mentorship with senior faculty or colleagues at other academic institutions to further career goals	Professional associations with group members; limited opportunities for career mentorship
6 Participation in hospital or departmental administration and policy is expected	Physician Autonomy

and bioinformatics, administrative support for faculty practice plans and medical education, and the complexity of managing the revenue streams of the 3 missions also contribute. Even when adjusted for a higher intensity case mix, AMC costs are 10% to 20% higher than community medical centers.[4]

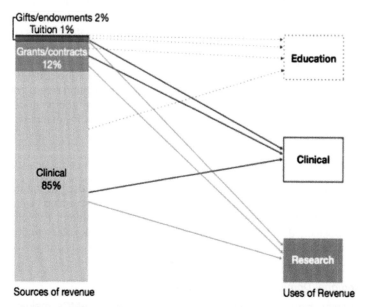

Fig. 2. Revenue cross-subsidization in academic medical centers. (*From* PwC Health Research Institute. The future of the academic medical center: strategies to avoid a margin meltdown. Available at: http://www.aahcdc.org/Portals/41/AIM-Program/Best-Practices/Financial_Alignment/The_Future_of_the_Academic_Medical_Center_Strategies_to_Avoid_Margin_Meltdown.pdf. Accessed October 1, 2017; with permission.)

ACADEMIC MEDICAL CENTERS IN THE NEW LANDSCAPE
Value-Based Care

Health care reform with a shift toward payment for value over volume does not favor the AMC model. Despite their strong reputations, AMCs as a group have not performed well on third-party quality rankings.[2] The highly specialized, high-cost care delivery models common in AMCs will present particular challenges in the changing marketplace. To compete in a value-based care world, AMCs may need to make significant changes to their care delivery systems. Focus is shifting toward primary preventive care models as opposed to specialized care, with an emphasis on creating more integrated provider networks. Primary care has not traditionally been a strong point for most AMCs, and capitated payment models are not likely to be favorable for institutions that serve a disproportionately high number of complicated, risky patients.

Many private health insurers are now creating narrow networks that favor providers and systems that demonstrate greater value; higher cost providers may be excluded. With their higher costs and limited quality upside to show for it, AMCs may find themselves left out of these plans. Given the higher reimbursements received from private insurers, AMCs cannot afford to lose this source of revenue.

Funding Threats

A confluence of factors mean that AMCs will face significant challenges to their financial viability, given their already precariously low operating margins.[5] AMCs are particularly vulnerable to changes in government funding across their 3 missions, and proposed changes to federal payment models may mean that as much as 10% of AMCs current funding sources are at risk.[2]

AMCs have a higher proportion of uninsured, Medicare, and Medicaid patients than non-AMCs, and they are projected to see an increase in their Medicare and Medicaid patient populations, and a decrease in privately insured patients (**Fig. 3**).[2] Government payors have significantly lower reimbursement rates than private insurers or self-pay patients.[6] Funding for the National Institutes of Health saw a decrease in funding capacity of 22% from 2003 to 2015, and although Congress increased the budget for 2016 and 2017, current levels are still well below what they were a decade ago in inflation-adjusted dollars.[7] Funding for graduate medical education is also in jeopardy, after a 2014 Medicare Payment Advisory Commission report recommended cuts in payments of up to 60%, based on findings that only 40% to 45% of indirect medical education payments were justified.[8]

DRIVERS FOR CONSOLIDATION

Many AMCs are facing an uncertain future and must either adapt to the new health care landscape or risk their survival. Pursuit of mergers or partnerships with community hospitals or health systems has been one way AMCs attempt to maintain their competitive position. Just as in any other industry, mergers take place to grow, diversify, and achieve economies of scale to achieve competitive advantage in a difficult market.

Achieve Regional Dominance and National Recognition

The high-acuity, high-complexity health care provided by AMCs makes them an attractive choice for many patients. AMCs are entering into strategic affiliations or mergers with community hospitals to further consolidate their regional dominance in multiple specialty services and become the preferred destination of choice for patients in the respective region. Interestingly, being viewed as a dominant regional health care

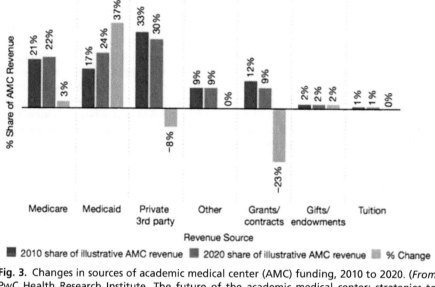

Fig. 3. Changes in sources of academic medical center (AMC) funding, 2010 to 2020. (*From* PwC Health Research Institute. The future of the academic medical center: strategies to avoid a margin meltdown. Available at: http://www.aahcdc.org/Portals/41/AIM-Program/Best-Practices/Financial_Alignment/The_Future_of_the_Academic_Medical_Center_Strategies_to_Avoid_Margin_Meltdown.pdf. Accessed October 1, 2017; with permission.)

provider further embellishes the national and international reputation of the AMCs, allowing further growth.

At the same time, community hospitals may feel competitive pressure to offer a wider range of services and specialty care than is truly justified by their case numbers. By combining forces, the complementary practices of academic and community hospitals would ideally lead to a system in which the strong primary care base provides consistent patient flow into specialized care when required, and patient care would become more integrated owing to taking place within the same system. Better stratification of patients to community or academic settings depending on their acuity and risk should lead to more appropriate care for the more high-risk patients who had previously been cared for in community settings, and lower cost care for low-risk patients who had been cared for in the academic setting.

Benefit from Economies of Scale

Mergers and partnerships in health care are undertaken with the idea that 1 benefit will be to achieve economies of scale, through decreasing both clinical and administrative overhead costs and enhanced purchasing and negotiating power. Industry research suggests potential cost savings of 15% to 30% from a successful merger.[9] Consolidation may also help to achieve other efficiencies beyond scale alone. Economies of scope, giving access to wider geographic and customer segments and economies of skill, allowing improved efficiencies in staffing and resource use and integration of care also create value if achieved.[10]

SHIFTING CONSOLIDATION MODELS

Although the Affordable Care Act and its move toward value-based care and bundled payments may be relatively new drivers in health care reform, a number of health care mergers occurred in the 1990s, in response to cuts to Medicare and pressure from managed care organizations.[11] The pace of mergers increased steadily in the mid-1990s, with approximately 750 hospital mergers occurring between 1994 and 1998. An analysis of 300 of those 750 concluded that the majority had been unsuccessful.[12]

Although academic–community mergers were successful, a number of high-profile failures including UCSF and Stanford, Penn State and Geisinger Healthy system, and NYU and Mt. Sinai have demonstrated the complexity of merging such large and established organizations. AMC–community mergers have taken many forms, from complete takeover via acquisition 1 one institution to full or partial business joint ventures involving the formation of a new separate parent company and bilateral equity contributions, to strategic alliances with varying degrees of equity involvement and maintenance of existing corporate structure.[10,11] In recent years, a shift from traditional full-scale mergers or acquisitions to non-mergers and acquisitions partnerships has occurred in consolidations involving AMCs, likely owing in large part to the financial constraints placed on AMC budgets by their affiliated universities, regulatory scrutiny, and credit downgrades impacting access to capital for asset based deals.[4,10]

CHALLENGES FACING ACADEMIC–COMMUNITY MERGERS

Despite the many promises of mergers and partnerships, a majority fail to realize their goals,[13] with some estimates going as far as a 90% failure rate.[14] Time and again, culture is cited as a key factor in the failure of mergers, both in health care and other industries.[12,15–18]

Culture: The Neglected Pitfall

With such robust evidence that culture is a "make-or-break factor in the merger equation,"[13] why is it so frequently ignored? Part of the problem may be in the difficulty in truly understanding organizational culture. With so many measurable, defined variables at play, the intangibles get left on the sidelines.

Understanding Culture in Organizations

Culture is integral to an organization, in much the same way as personality is to an individual,[13] and it encompasses a number of different features (**Fig. 4**). Members of a particular group are connected through one or more such elements that define their culture, and these elements become a core part of their identity. It is difficult to assess a priori the potential for culture clash in a merger. Further, mergers become incredibly difficult to manage once a culture clash takes root. People are hesitant to alter established behaviors and practices because any change is often perceived as a loss.

Layers of organizational culture

Although an organization may cite its mission statement as a representation of its underlying culture, this may not be accurate, according to Schein's theory of layered organizational culture.[12] Institutions with similar mission statements may interpret

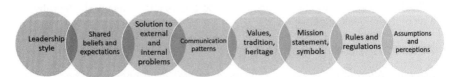

Fig. 4. Defining organizational culture.

them in very different ways as a result of their disparate values and assumptions as well as their heritage and traditions. In analyzing the failure of the merger between Pennsylvania State University's Hershey Medical Center and Geisinger Health System, culture came up numerous times as a reason for failure, despite the fact that their cultural similarities were initially cited as a major predictor of their compatibility.[12] Although both had mission statements citing patient care, education, and research as core features, they failed to recognize that their priorities differed significantly with regard to the deeper levels of understanding and executing that mission.

Competing values

Another method for evaluating organizational cultures is the competing values framework (CVF).[19] This framework describes 2 dimensions along which an organizations values are measured, one being the locus of control (centralized, highly controlled compared with decentralized, more flexible) and the other being focus on internal environment and process compared with a focus on external environment or relationships (**Fig. 5**). The CVF is the most commonly used cultural assessment tool used in the health care industry, and is generally considered to be well-validated and reliable; caution must be applied in generalizing results to populations in which it has not been validated.[20] Within the health care literature, the CVF has been validated only among managers,[21] despite being applied to nonmanager employees in numerous studies. The CVF has been used to demonstrate the impact of organizational culture on patient satisfaction,[22] employee job satisfaction,[23] safety,[24] and hospital

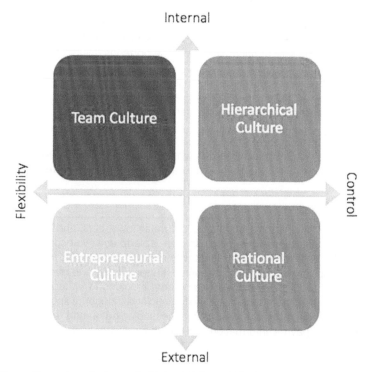

Fig. 5. Competing values framework. (*Adapted from* Helfrich CD, Li YF, Mohr DC, et al. Assessing an organizational culture instrument based on the Competing Values Framework: Exploratory and confirmatory factor analyses. Implement Sci 2007;2(1):13; with permission.)

performance.[25] Echoing findings of the layered model of culture, application of the CVF to a cohort of academic physicians employed at both a teaching institution and its partner local health system found that although both had overlapping missions, their organizational cultures differed substantially.[26] The distinction between the culture of the academic and the clinical sites led to challenges a few years later when they were merged into a new trust.[15]

Communication

Cultural clashes result in deteriorating communication, and worsening collaboration and coordination with reduced productivity within the new organization. "Conversation is a determinant and not just an outcome of culture,"[27] and is therefore inextricably linked with the cultural challenges merging organizations face. Applying the metaphor of marriage to mergers, the vital role of effective communication becomes evident. By understanding communication patterns, organizations may be better able to predict the chances of success in a merger, and better equipped to intervene effectively if the change process struggles.

Leadership

Leadership and organizational culture are inextricably linked,[18] and leaders need to recognize and address cultural factors to guide their organizations through a merger or other major change in structure. The power struggles within the leadership can lead to a lack of direction and confusion among the staff, ultimately causing a reduced commitment to mission and goals. Differences in management style between two merging organizations can cause problems, as can a lack of alignment between the leadership driving the mergers and the physicians and other clinical staff who are "on the ground." In this environment, those who are dissatisfied and disaffected leave the organization. The loss of talent and expertise portends failure of the merger.

It is imperative that leadership maintains the trust of the organization, and in some cases the secretive nature of merger discussions, perceived as reflective of "corporate culture," serves to undermine the success of the change process, which tends to be more collaborative and open in academic culture.[12]

Other Challenges

Operational and financial challenges can worsen cultural clashes. When merging organizations fail to see the gains they had anticipated, cultural differences can be magnified.

Theoretic Versus Realized Economies

Larger size alone for a health system does not mean lower cost, and in fact one study found that although stand-alone hospitals were able to achieve economies of scale, this was not the case for health systems with multiple facilities.[9] This may be due in large part to failure to consolidate personnel, support staff, and overhead costs, as well as difficulty setting system-wide standards, resulting in all facilities continuing to operate essentially independently. A systematic and thoughtful approach is needed to achieve for the integration of various services including human resource management, finance and payroll, information and technology, supply chain, or staffing.

Brand Dilution

One of an AMC's most significant assets may be its brand and name recognition. Partnering with community health systems risks diluting this brand and undermining the benefits of consolidation for both parties. Community hospitals and private practice groups may also face a change in their public perception, if merging with a large AMC is perceived as detrimental to the more personal, community-based feel of the organization.

Impacts of Consolidation on Anesthesia Groups

As with the larger health systems they are a part of, academic and private practice anesthesiology groups can differ substantially and will face specific challenges in combining their workforces and workflow. Consolidation of anesthesia groups will most often occur in the context of a merger or partnership of their parent organizations, and both system-wide and specialty-specific factors will affect the success of combining different practice models. Beyond the drivers for consolidation discussed previously, partnerships involving academic and private practice anesthesia groups may realize the benefits enumerated in **Box 2**.

Productivity and Efficiency

Differences in compensation plans and productivity metrics may cause complexity in merging academic and community anesthesia groups, because in general academic anesthesiologists earn lower salaries than those in the community, but their income is not based solely on billable units and clinical work. Disparate workflows and practice models involving other anesthesia providers may also lead to a bumpy integration process. If the two disparate practices cannot be kept on separate practice and

---

Box 2
Benefits of a merger/partnership to community private practice and academic anesthesiology groups

Benefits to Community Private Practice Groups	Benefits to Academic Anesthesiology Groups
Income and employment security	Opportunity to achieve more efficient management of resources and staff
Access to better employee benefits (retirement, health, disability, etc) at a lower cost	Improved risk stratification with more appropriate distribution of cases based on hospital resources
Size-related cost efficiencies and purchasing power	Access to large pools of patients for research
Leveraged negotiating with payers and health systems	Expand primary and secondary care base for referrals
Opportunity for increased income based on performance incentives and/or better use of staff, CRNAs, and AAs	Provide different clinical experience for trainees
Management infrastructure, OR management expertise	Enhanced integration of primary and surgical/anesthesia care
Investment in information technology and data collection/analysis	Access to broader geographic area
Access to risk management, quality management and compliance programs	Understanding of private practice management and entrepreneurial skills
Educational opportunities for new faculty members	Opportunity for trainees to learn in new practice settings
Leadership and career development and mentorship opportunities	
Implementation of evidence-based standardized protocols and best practices	

Abbreviations: AA, anesthesia assistant; CRNA, certified registered nurse anesthetist; OR, operating room.

compensation plans that allow maximum productivity and fair compensation for serviced provide, then new compensation schemes will need to be formulated. When merging, it is important to recognize the value of preserving the key elements of practice that make both AMCs and community private practices successful in their goals.

Academic Mission

Research and education are core components of an academic anesthesiology group's mission and can be major factors in a cultural divide between merging organizations. Academic anesthesiologists are expected to spend a portion of their time performing "nonclinical" duties, including teaching residents and medical students, basic science and clinical research, and quality improvement initiatives. Although some anesthesiologists in private practice groups may be motivated and enjoy engaging in some of these additional activities, that is unlikely to be the case across the board. Anesthesiologists may have selected their practice based on their own preferences and desire to avoid any teaching or research responsibilities and coming under the umbrella of an academic group may cause significant friction if all members of the group are expected to function as academic faculty.

Impact When Merging Residency Programs

Although no literature on mergers of anesthesia training programs exists, similar experiences from other specialties can inform the effects on residents when an academic and community-based program are merged. In one survey of pediatric residents after a merger, perceptions differed dramatically depending on which program the trainees started in.[28] Overall, those who started in the community program had positive feedback on the merger's impact on their educational experience and on the institutions as a whole. The impact of differences in race, ethnicity, and culture on the dynamics of the new combined program was also noted as an unexpected challenge when combining the 2 programs. Surgical residents who started in a community program that subsequently merged with an academic program reported positive effects on clinical education, didactics, and career opportunities.[29] Despite these upsides, the same cohort also noted negative impact on relational metrics, including feeling less like part of a team, a decrease in the strength of their support system, and no longer feeling that their program was like a family. Another survey on surgical residencies reported an overall positive perception among both residents on faculty on the case mix and academic atmosphere, but a negative impact on morale, relationships between residency and faculty, and hospital support.[30] Based on the experience of residency mergers in Boston, Rider and Longmaid[31] outlined guidelines to smooth the process, the majority of which involved cultural or interpersonal factors that needed to be addressed. Despite varied responses on the educational impact of residency mergers, the impact on cultural and relational metrics are consistently reported as major challenges, reflecting the experience of the overarching institutional merger.

SUMMARY

Mergers and partnerships involving AMCs and community practices are likely inevitable in the current landscape. Past experience has shown that there is no one "right" model for consolidation to achieve guaranteed success, but that does not mean there is nothing to be learned from those successes and failures. Health systems contemplating consolidation must look at the same metrics and perform the same due diligence as would be expected of any other multimillion-dollar organizations in other industries.

REFERENCES

1. Association of American Medical Colleges (AAMC). What roles do teaching hospitals fulfill? Available at: https://www.aamc.org/download/54360/data/whatrolesdothfulfill. pdf. Accessed October 12, 2017.
2. Health Research Institute. The future of the academic medical center: Strategies to avoid a margin meltdown. Price Watershouse Cooper (PWC) [white paper]; 2012. Available at: https://www.pwc.com/us/en/health-industries/health-research-institute/ publications/pdf/the-future-of-academic-medical-centers.pdf. Accessed October 3, 2017.
3. Institute of Medicine. Graduate medical education that meets the nation's health needs. Washington, DC: The National Academies Press; 2014.
4. Deloitte Center for Health Solutions. Academic medical centers: the tipping point. 2007. Available at: www.deloitte.com/us/amctippingpoint. Accessed October 7, 2017.
5. Kutscher B. Hospitals, systems see operating margins shrink as expenses climb. Modern Healthcare; 2014. Available at: http://www.modernhealthcare.com/ article/20140813/NEWS/308139963. Accessed November 9, 2017.
6. Wan W, Itri J, Cross B. Charge master: friend or foe? Curr Probl Diagn Radiol 2016;45:122–7.
7. NIH Research Funding Trends. Federation of American Societies for Experimental Biology. Available at: http://faseb.org/Science-Policy–Advocacy-and-Communications/Federal-Funding-Data/NIH-Research-Funding-Trends.aspx. Accessed November 9, 2017.
8. Fleishon HB, Itri JN, Boland GW, et al. Academic medical centers and community hospitals integration: trends and strategies. J Am Coll Radiol 2017;14(1):45–51.
9. Mohr J, Pilgrim G, Bales T, et al. Size should matter: Five ways to help healthcare systems realize the benefits of scale. PwC Strategy & [White paper] 2016. Available at: https://www.strategyand.pwc.com/reports/size-should-matter. Accessed October 12, 2017.
10. Harris A, Kumar P, Sutaria S. Unlocking the potential of academic and community health system partnerships. 2015. Available at: http://healthcare.mckinsey.com/ sites/default/files/AMC partnerships %28McK white paper%29.pdf. Accessed October 1, 2017.
11. Cohen MD, Jennings G. Mergers involving academic medical institutions: impact on academic radiology departments. J Am Coll Radiol 2005;2(2):174–82.
12. Mallon WT. The alchemists: a case study of a failed merger in academic medicine. Acad Med 2003;78(11):1090–104.
13. Schraeder M, Self DR. Enhancing the success of mergers and acquisitions: an organizational culture perspective. Manag Decis 2003;41(5):511–22.
14. Martin RL. M&A: the one thing you need to get right. Harv Bus Rev 2016;5(5):42–8.
15. Ovseiko PV, Melham K, Fowler J, et al. Organisational culture and post-merger integration in an academic health centre: a mixed-methods study. BMC Health Serv Res 2015;15(1):25.
16. Belokrinitsky I, McCann C. 5 pitfalls to avoid in managing the cultural aspect of health system integration. Becker's Hospital Review. 2015. Available at: https:// www.beckershospitalreview.com/hospital-management-administration/5-pitfalls-to-avoid-in-managing-the-cultural-aspect-of-health-system-integration.html?tmpl= component&print=1&layout=default&page=. Accessed November 9, 2017.
17. Thier SO, Kelley WN, Pardes H, et al. Success factors in merging teaching hospitals. Acad Med 2014;89(2):219–23.

18. Bligh MC. Surviving post-merger "culture clash": can cultural leadership lessen the casualties? Leadership 2006;2(4):395–426.
19. Quinn RE, Rohrbaugh J. A competing values approach to organizational effectiveness. Public Product Rev 1981;5(2):122–40.
20. Helfrich CD, Li Y-F, Mohr DC, et al. Assessing an organizational culture instrument based on the competing values framework: exploratory and confirmatory factor analyses. Implement Sci 2007;2(1):13.
21. Kalliath T, Bluedorn A, Gillespie D. A confirmatory factor analysis of the competing values instrument. Educ Psychol Meas 1999;59(1):143–58.
22. Meterko M, Mohr DC, Young GJ. Teamwork culture and patient satisfaction in hospitals. Med Care 2004;42:492–8.
23. Zazzali JL, Alexander JA, Shortell SM, et al. Organizational culture and physician satisfaction with dimensions of group practice. Health Serv Res 2007;42:1150–76.
24. Hartmann CW, Meterko M, Rosen AK. Relationship of hospital organizational culture to patient safety climate in the Veterans Health Administration. Med Care Res Rev 2009;66:320–38.
25. Jacobs R, Mannion R, Davies HTO, et al. The relationship between organizational culture and performance in acute hospitals. Soc Sci Med 2013;76:115–25.
26. Ovseiko PV, Buchan AM. Organizational culture in an academic health center. Acad Med 2012;87(6):709–18.
27. Dooley KJ, Zimmerman BJ. Merger as marriage: communication issues in post-merger integration. Health Care Manage Rev 2003;28(1):55–67.
28. Cora-bramble D, Joseph J, Jain S, et al. A cross-cultural pediatric residency program merger. Acad Med 2006;81(12):1108–14.
29. Tackett JJ, Longo WE, Lebastchi AH, et al. Combining disparate surgical residencies into one: lessons learned. J Surg Res 2015;198(2):289–93.
30. Mellinger J, Bonnell B, Passinault W, et al. Resident and faculty perceptions of a surgical residency program merger. Curr Surg 2001;58(2):223–6.
31. Rider EA, Longmaid HE. A model for merging residency programmes during health care consolidations: a course for success. Med Educ 2003;37(9):794–801.

Moving?

Make sure your subscription moves with you!

To notify us of your new address, find your **Clinics Account Number** (located on your mailing label above your name), and contact customer service at:

Email: journalscustomerservice-usa@elsevier.com

800-654-2452 (subscribers in the U.S. & Canada)
314-447-8871 (subscribers outside of the U.S. & Canada)

Fax number: 314-447-8029

Elsevier Health Sciences Division
Subscription Customer Service
3251 Riverport Lane
Maryland Heights, MO 63043

*To ensure uninterrupted delivery of your subscription, please notify us at least 4 weeks in advance of move.

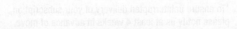

Printed and bound by CPI Group (UK) Ltd, Croydon, CR0 4YY

12/05/2025

01866958-0001